EXECUTIVE HEALTH

A BusinessWeek Book

EXECUTIVE HEALTH

how to recognize
health danger signals
and manage stress successfully
by Philip Goldberg

First paperback edition, 1979
Library of Congress Cataloging in Publication Data

Goldberg, Philip.
    Executive health.

    1. Executives—Health programs. 2. Stess
(Physiology) I. Title. [DNLM: 1. Administrative
personnel—Popular works. 2. Mental health—
Popular works. 3. Stress, Psychological—Popular
works. WM172 G618e]
RA778.5.G65   613   78-5969
ISBN 0-07-023647-X
ISBN 0-07-023638-0 (paperback)

     4 5 6 7 8 9 0 DODO   8 3 2 1

Editorial production services provided by Cobb/Dunlop, Inc.
Printed in the United States of America.

contents

introduction

I am tempted to look at this book as a thesaurus on stress in organizational life. A good deal has been written about the stressor effect of executive responsibilities in middle and top management, but unfortunately, very few of these publications are of any direct use to the people being studied. Therefore it is most encouraging that Philip Goldberg has filled the void with an extremely practical, useful guide for present-day executives.

The author's ideas run virtually parallel to my own, as expressed in my small book STRESS WITHOUT DISTRESS, although I must add that his volume is of far greater value to the executive. My booklet discussing the stress concept in general for the layman received much more attention from executives and management than I had anticipated. Since its publication in 1974 and the creation of our International Institute of Stress in 1977, occupational stress has become a major category in our Library and Documentation Center, a collection of more than 120,000 publications on stress and stress-related topics. We are now constantly receiving requests from executive personnel for more and more information on the topic. EXECUTIVE HEALTH answers this need by being a very timely and necessary handbook for this specialized group of people.

This book is a rich collection of quotes by contemporary experts on stress and stress management. It gives brief but clear descriptions of the most common stressors in daily life. The range of subjects discussed is broad enough to provide a sound comprehension of the stress concept in all its complexities. Cardiovascular diseases, hypertension, atherosclerosis, peptic ulcers, migraine headaches, diabetes, and cancer are described in easily understandable terms, followed by an examination of the most common causes of these maladies and their treatments.

Although primarily written for the executive, I feel certain that the volume offers most useful information to any physician, especially to psychiatrists, but also to psychologists, ethologists, and to the educated reading public at large. I would hope that, besides helping the individual reader, it would bring about much-needed changes in company policies concerning employee health. The trend toward reducing occupational stress has begun gaining momentum in some of the more progressive American companies, yet the overall industrial picture of North America is not very encouraging. Much more care and attention needs to be given to introducing and maintaining higher health standards of employees.

It would seem somewhat impertinent for a physician to make such a suggestion, but I do not think that it is an unreasonable one for, as this book amply demonstrates, industry suffers stupendous losses because of excessive occupational stresses culminating in absenteeism, alcoholism, drug abuse on the job, early mortality, and so forth. I am even inclined to think that the available statistics underestimate the actual financial losses which in all probability remain hidden because of improper functioning and mismanagement of human resources and energy.

In my own—unfortunately too infrequent—personal contacts with executives, businessmen, managers, and other top-level employees, I have noticed their growing concern about the debilitating effects of excessive stress on the job which carries over into their personal lives. Some of my encounters with these individuals have been a source of much distress to me, for it is most difficult to explain that the solution to their problems lies not in tranquilizers and other prescription drugs, but in such preventive measures as a more healthy and reasonable attitude towards life in general and work in particular, proper diet, exercise and relaxation, reinforced by a more natural code of behavior. Anyone can be his own best physician once he has understood the mechanisms of stress and determined his own level of stress tolerance.

Philip Goldberg's EXECUTIVE HEALTH questions the implicit trust placed in medicine as a cure-all for stress diseases. It puts the onus of being healthy squarely on the shoulders of the individual. Its directives are clear: in the final analysis, no one can look after us better than we ourselves. But it does not stop there: it provides a simplified but necessary health program for industry that would benefit not only executives and management personnel but also lower-echelon employees. It should be an invaluable handbook to one and all, also because it provides a detailed listing of existing stress clinics and institutes whose facilities and services would supplement, if necessary, the stress reduction techniques advocated by the author.

The wisdom of today's spiritual movements and physical fitness institutions is examined closely since these are the present adaptation measures occupying mankind at present. They are being explored from different directions but all become centered around the wellbeing of the human organism.

Man is a working animal whose mental and physical qualities must be employed sufficiently for him to remain healthy and prevent emotional as well as physical atrophy. But he must also learn to recognize that sometimes his work is so consuming that it robs him of the ability to develop in other areas of his being.

The research done on executive populations is here compiled and made available so that the final product is a sound outline of what every executive can do to improve himself and live a much more rewarding life. The enthusiasm instilled by these recommendations is exhilarating. We every so often need to refresh our confidence that stress can indeed be mastered.

> *Hans Selye, C.C., M.D., Ph.D., D.Sc.*
> *President*
> *International Institute of Stress*
> *Montreal, Quebec*
> *April 28, 1978*

preface

Health is becoming as important a subject in boardrooms and executive suites as salaries, taxes, or the cost of depreciation. Indeed, depreciation is an appropriate metaphor; health—both physical and mental—legitimately concerns corporations because it strongly influences the performance of the most vital piece of equipment a company can possess—the human being.

American companies have increasingly assumed responsibility for the health and happiness of employees. In recent years, in-house medical and psychiatric programs have proliferated, as have company-sponsored conferences, retreats, gymnasiums, meditation rooms, and other health-related programs, including imaginative excursions like the Menninger Foundation's growth seminars conducted on white-water canoeing expeditions.

Why the increasing concern? Is it a response to the public demand for corporate responsibility? Is it simply a reflection of the post-1960s preoccupation with the quality of life? Is health-promotion cost-effective? Clearly, the dollars and cents impact of health problems, and the growing understanding of how they can be caused or aggravated by the work environment, have stirred businessmen to action. At the bottom line, health cannot be ignored, nor can affirmative action be delayed:

- *Premature employee death costs American industry $19.4 billion a year, more than the combined 1976 profits of Fortune's top five corporations.*
- *An estimated $10 to $20 billion is lost through absence, hospitalization, and early death among executives.*
- *Alcoholism costs industry about $15.6 billion annually due to absenteeism and medical costs.*
- *About 32 million workdays, and $8.6 billion in wages is lost annually to heart-related diseases.*
- *According to the American Heart Association, the cost of recruiting replacements for executives felled by heart disease is about $700 million a year.*

If we add to those figures the lost skills, experience, contacts, and wisdom of executives whose careers are cut short, and the diminished effectiveness of managers plagued by nagging maladies and emotional upsets, the cost soars beyond calculation. Truly, human intelligence and energy are our most vital resources. Realizing that, executives are beginning to invest heavily in their own and their employees' health.

In recognition of this trend, Business Week decided to publish a comprehensive guide to executive health, the purpose of which is three-fold:

- *to give businesspeople a basic understanding of the sources and symptoms of the ailments to which they are particularly vulnerable—those associated with a high-stress lifestyle.*
- *to let them know what their peers and health experts are thinking and doing about those problems.*
- *most important, to provide them with a multidimensional battery of effective methods for safeguarding health and managing stress.*

new trends in health

In researching this book, we discovered a health-care world in transition. Old notions and treatment procedure have been called into question as a new generation of health professionals realized that Americans are not quite as healthy as we all thought. Advances in medical technology have largely wiped out the infectious diseases that plagued our ancestors, but a host of new disorders has spread to epidemic proportions. Cardiovascular disease, cancer, stroke, and other big killers are relatively new; only three instances of cardiac arrest appeared in the medical literature before this century. While more people avoid death in their early years now, the average white male of 50 years can reasonably expect to live to age 73, only 9 months longer than his counterpart in the 1920s.

The medical field is bursting with imaginative research, astounding technology, and bold, far-reaching ideas. Predictably, controversy abounds. Theories and counter-theories—each seemingly supported by ample data—compete with one another, and few unequivocal answers are available to key questions.

As we pored through the literature and interviewed the experts, several trends became discernible. While they have not yet attracted the entire medical community, it seems evident that these trends herald a bright new orientation toward health. The new emphasis centers upon the following areas.

Natural treatment

The dangerous and unforseen side effects of drugs, and the fact that they tend to merely mask symptoms without removing the underlying cause, have swayed medical experts toward a more cautious approach to medication. Reports of unnecessary, and often harmful, operations have similarly affected attitudes toward surgery. Alternatives are recommended when possible, and research on drugless therapies is increasing.

Prevention

Traditionally, Western medicine has focused on intervention—the treatment of illness once it has manifested to the point where symptoms are evident. All too often, this crisis-oriented approach has left the door open for a return of symptoms or the development of new ones; neither does intervention necessarily promote *good* health, in spite of successfully removing some pathology. As a result, the emphasis has been shifting to identification of disease in its primitive stages, thus enabling physicians to correct problems before they become pathological.

But now, even preventive medicine is giving way to still newer concepts reminiscent of the ancient Chinese custom of paying a village physician to keep every one well, and docking him if someone took ill. The notion of health as a state of mental and physical perfection, as opposed to merely being *not sick,* has taken hold. Terms such as "promotive medicine" appear increasingly in health writing, and especially the term "wellness."

The trend is mirrored in the mental health field, where the old Freudian mode of treating recognizable neurosis and psychosis has largely been supplanted by the school of humanistic psychology. Spurred by the research of pioneering psychologist Abraham Maslow, this approach emphasizes the promotion of self-actualization and human potential.

"It is as if Freud supplied us with the sick half of psychology, and we must now fill in the healthy half," wrote Maslow. "Perhaps this health psychology will give us more possibility of controlling and improving our lives and for making ourselves better people. Perhaps this will be more fruitful than asking 'how to get unsick.'"

Patient Responsibility

While it has long been known that the patient's attitude plays a considerable role in his responsiveness to treatment, it is only recently that physicians are turning over a major share of responsibility to the patient. "People assume more responsibility for the welfare of their cars than their own bodies," deplores one physician. "If they helped themselves more, we wouldn't need as many hospitals."

Becoming healthy, and remaining so, means more than seeing a doctor when we get sick. It means becoming aware of the precursors of illness, and doing those things that promote health, while refraining from those that damage it.

Holistic Health

"Since the Middle Ages," writes psychologist Ken Pelletier, author of *Mind as Healer, Mind as Slayer,* "Western philosophers have divided man into the separate aspects of body, mind, and spirit. We in the West think in terms of these parts of man rather than seeing him as an integrated whole. This split is evident in the present division of the healing professions. Physicians treat the body; psychologists and psychiatrists heal the mind; and yet a third group, the clergy, attends to the soul."

Recognizing this historical shortcoming, the healing sciences are expanding their procedures to include all aspects of a person's life. We are complex organisms composed of a multitude of elements—physical, mental, emotional, environmental—that come together interdependently to create something greater than a collection of parts. Each area of life influences the others, and the boundaries between causes and effects blur and shift continuously.

Thus, modern clinics are becoming increasingly interdisciplinary. Physicians from all areas of specialization are being joined by psychologists, who also have their specialties, and by nutritionists, physiotherapists, experts in relaxation, exercise, lifestyle, and various natural healing procedures, in a massive assault on disease and a concerted thrust toward health.

This book attempts to comply with these new trends. It describes the nature of disease-causing stress. It brings you the most highly regarded self-care procedures for prevention, and in some cases, treatment of stress disorders, as well as guidelines for obtaining professional aid. These are approached from all angles, in keeping with the holistic orientation of today's authorities.

Making the most of the book may require candid evaluation of your personality, habits, values, and attitudes. To aid you in achieving the necessary insight a number of self-evaluative questionnaires have been included. Without personal contact with an expert, and without the use of highly sophisticated measuring instruments, precise quantification of health-related variables is, of course, impossible. However, these informal aids to introspection can help you locate your problem areas and decide which procedures you should adopt to raise your level of physical, mental, and emotional perfection.

Philip Goldberg

February 1978
New York City

acknowledgements

First and foremost, I wish to thank Lincoln Platt, director of new product development at Business Week, who helped conceive this project and set the tone of the book, and who deserves special credit for seeing that it got done. Deep appreciation to Christine Larson-Turner and Steven Cohen of the Business Week staff; Peggy Tsukahira, consulting editor from McGraw-Hill books; Allen Cobb, Bob Goldberg, and Jane Brodie, for their assistance in researching and editing the book.

We would like to thank all the professional men and women who lent us their time and expertise: Carmen Moynehan, Dr. Benjamin Natovitz, and Dr. John A. Rossa of Executive Health Examiners; Dolores R. Floss and Dr. Charles M. Ross of Life Extension Institute; Nathan Pritikin and Robert Palmer of Longevity Center; Dr. Sidney Lecker and Dr. Howard Glazer of Stress Control Systems Inc.; Dr. Rosalind Forbes, Dr. Meyer Friedman, Dr. Harold Bloomfield, Dr. Carl Thoreson, Dr. Elliot Goldwag, Charles Swencionis, Lynn Krown, John Kiley, Dr. Barry Charles, Samuel Bursuk, Barbara MacNeil, Dr. John Travis, Jim Donahue, Stu Mooney, Dr. Mardi Horowitz, Dr. Bernard Glueck, Dr. David Frew, Richard Grossman, Sally Nelson, Don Isbell, Christopher Hegerty, and Bill Gilbertson.

Special thanks to Dr. Hans Selye, for his introduction, and for paving the way to a deeper understanding of stress.

executive stress

the challenge of the twentieth century

We have left undone those things which we ought to have done; And we have done those things which we ought not to have done; And there is no health in us.——*The Book of Common Prayer*

the town that was immune to stress

Roseto, Pennsylvania was founded by Italian immigrants in the 1880s and maintained the old way of life for 80 years. The men worked in nearby slate quarries and the women maintained the home, just as their ancestors had done for generations. The families were tightly knit and raised their children according to traditional values. Meals were the high points of each day, with ample wine and fatty meats. Yet, despite high-cholesterol diets and a tendency toward overweight, the death rate was remarkably low—the incidence of heart disease was one-third the national average and only one-fourth that of Roseto's neighboring towns. No citizen under 47 years of age had ever had a heart attack. For that reason, Roseto became known as "Miracle Town."

That was in 1961. Ten years later, Dr. John G. Bruhn of the University of Texas returned to Roseto and was astonished at what he found. In a decade, the town had become modernized. The men now commuted to out-of-town jobs. The teenagers were going far away to college. Cars choked the thoroughfares of the village. T.V. antennas sprouted from rooftops like grapes from old-country vines. Families ate on the run. And the incidence of heart disease climbed up to the expected rate.

"In Roseto," wrote Dr. Bruhn at the time, "family and community support is disappearing. Most of the men who have had heart attacks here were living under stress and really had nowhere to turn to relieve that pressure. . . . These people have given up something, and it's killing them."

—————————————— social sources of stress ——————

What the citizens of Roseto did in a decade, the rest of us have done in not much longer. Two hundred years ago—a wink in biological time —the population of the United States was 3,930,000—about half the current population of New Jersey. Only 202,000 (less than 5 percent) lived in towns and villages of more than 2500. "We are not used to a complicated civilization," wrote Walter Lippman. "We have changed our environment more quickly than we know how to change ourselves." Nor has physical evolution had sufficient time to equip us with the best psychological apparatus to maximize successful adaptation.

Disease represents a failure of the organism to adapt to some potentially destructive influence. Accordingly, every epoch has had its characteristic maladies: the Middle Ages had the plague, the Renaissance had syphilis, the Romantic Era had tuberculosis. The advent of an industrialized, urban way of life has given rise to a host of new disorders. In a sense, we have created a mixed blessing—unprecedented prosperity and universal access to comforts and culture, at the expense of a milieu that is wreaking havoc with our bodies and severely limiting our ability to enjoy our hard-earned affluence. An estimated 80 percent of all modern disease has its origins in what has come to be called *stress*.

Research supports the notion that changing life-styles can contribute to illness. According to Dr. Leonard Syme of the University of California School of Public Health, men whose life situation is different from that in which they grew up run an increased risk of heart attack. For example, a farm boy who moves to the big city and takes a white-collar job increases his risk by 300 percent. If he takes a blue-collar job, the risk increases far less radically. Differences in diet, amount of physical activity, weight, and age do not, according to Dr. Syme, account for the difference.

Modern man is beseiged by more unrelenting pressures and rapid-fire stimulation than at any time in history. The result is not only the celebrated forms of neurosis and alienation that social scientists have chronicled, but numerous crippling diseases spurned by an overload on the body's adaptive mechanisms. "There is absolutely no question that one can overshoot the stimulation of the endocrine system," states noted biologist Dr. René Dubos. "This has physiological consequences that last throughout the whole lifetime of the organism."

In the pages that follow, we shall survey the variety of modern social and environmental changes that have so suddenly become vital issues in modern life. As we shall see, important new forces affecting the health and well-being of society come from a dozen different directions. Although these forces are often clearly definable, they are perhaps more often diffused throughout the whole fabric of daily life. The very notion of health, therefore, has become as broad and diversified as human potential itself. We are forced to concern ourselves with the *holistic* value of health, which stretches all the way from what we eat to how we think, and to the very quality of life.

change

Perhaps the most significant change that modern man faces is change itself—rapid, unpredictable, or disorienting change. Alvin Toffler, whose exhaustively documented book, *Future Shock,* has become a modern classic, provides a brilliant but disturbing picture of civilization bombarded by incessant change. Says Toffler: "There are discoverable limits to the amount of change that the human organism can absorb. . . . By endlessly accelerating change without first determining these limits, we may submit masses of men to demands they simply cannot tolerate."

Some changes, of course, are more damaging than others. Some are not damaging at all: they are life enhancing. What is clear is that change of any kind places demands on us, mentally and physically. Too much change can wear us out. Precisely how that occurs will be discussed in subsequent chapters. Here we shall describe some of the more significant changes to which humankind has been newly subjected.

Crowding

"In all species experimentally investigated," writes Dr. Hudson Hoagland, "the mortality is found to be dependent on population density and to cease below a certain critical population density." Animal studies suggest that population control may be an instinctive behavior pattern.

stress of crowding

In 1916, five deer were released on James Island in Chesapeake Bay, a territory of half a square mile. In 1956, 300 deer were added. Two years later, over half were dead. The death rate continued into the following year and finally leveled off at 80. Was it, as Thomas Malthus

> might have insisted, a shortage of food that caused the population to dwindle? Apparently not—there was an adequate food supply, and the density never exceeded one deer per acre of land. An examination of the dead deer showed that their adrenal glands were 81 percent heavier than normal. Adrenals are the only glands that enlarge under stress.

Studies have been performed on mice, rabbits, and other animals, all with the same results—wholesale death despite adequate food supplies, and, upon autopsy, evidence of severe stress disorders. Can this explain the bizarre mass suicide of well-fed lemmings who plunge helter-skelter into the Arctic Ocean?

Studies of primitive tribes suggest a theory of "optimum numbers" for humans, too. Apparently, populations fluctuate only slightly around a fixed figure, which is sustained by such acts as infanticide, compulsory abortion, cannibalism, head-hunting, sacrifice, ritual murder, and numerous taboos.

Is crowding itself the impetus behind such phenomena? Are crowds, as such, really unhealthy, or do other factors intervene? Scientists are so far puzzled.

Reactions to crowds apparently vary from one culture to the next. The French, Italians, Greeks, Arabs, and Japanese, for example, have a higher tolerance than the English, Germans, Scandinavians, and Americans. Hong Kong has one of the highest population densities in the world, yet, with the exception of tuberculosis, disease rates are relatively low, mortality rates are two-thirds that of the United States, and hospitalization for mental illness is a tenth that of the United States.

Noise

It has long been known that excessive noise can erode hearing; an estimated 18 million Americans have some hearing loss attributable to exposure to noise. Now we have evidence that noise—especially loud, meaningless, irregular, and unpredictable noise—can also damage performance, behavior, and mental health.

A classic study on the effects of noise was performed by psychologists David Glass and Jerome Singer, at a 32-story apartment building rising directly above a twelve-lane highway in a major American city. Over a four-year period the researchers gathered data on the children living in the building. Those on the lower floors had impaired learning abilities. Especially blemished was their ability to make subtle discriminations between similar-sounding words. The researchers concluded that the children had to make a subconscious effort to filter out noise, and had thus screened out distinctions important to learning.

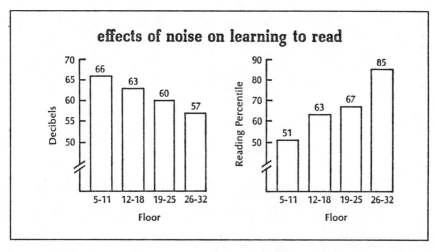

In another study, the researchers used galvanic skin response, a reliable indicator of arousal in the autonomic nervous system. They found that noise of all degrees of loudness and unpredictability increased stress, even when the individual's mind was able to "block it out." Immediately after removing the source of noise, the galvanic skin response returned to normal. The subjects were then given puzzles to solve. The group that had not been exposed to noise earlier did significantly better than the ones who were. Significantly, the noise's unpredictability was more detrimental to subsequent performance than its loudness. The group exposed to soft, unpredictable noise performed worse than the group exposed to loud but predictable noise.

decibel counts of common noise producers

Research indicates that the annoyance threshold is 50 to 90 decibels, and that the threshold of actual pain is 120 decibels:

Vacuum cleaner	81 decibels
Sports car or truck	90
Blenders	93
Pneumatic jackhammer	94
Outboard motors	102
Loud power motor	107
Group of electric guitars	114
Riveter	130
Jet plane on ьakeoff	150

At sounds above 70 decibels (about the noise level of a relatively quiet city street) the autonomic nervous system begins to become aroused—often without the individual even becoming aware of it. In addition to impaired performance, hormonal changes probably occur, which could lead to physical and mental difficulties.

Interestingly, control over the noise makes a big difference in its impact. The sounds of a typewriter, for example, will disturb an executive's performance more when the typist is *someone else's* secretary rather than his own.

---

stress of noise

The World Health Organization estimates that illness and impairment due to noise has cost the world's industries over $4 billion. Studies show that on-the-job noise can create the following problems:

permanent hearing loss
increased heart and circulatory problems
equilibrium disturbance
digestive disorders
diminished job performance
increased accident rates
increased absenteeism.

Air Pollution

Environmentalists have long warned us of the lung damage caused by polluted city air. More recent findings show that the degree of human alertness, vigilance, and ability to perform simple addition and sentence comprehension all decline under polluted conditions. These findings have important implications for business and industry; even commuters breathe in large amounts of carbon monoxide getting to and from the office.

Dr. Steven M. Horvath writes that "CO (carbon monoxide), a component of polluted air, [is] capable of impairing various complex psychophysiological functions." He adds that persons with high exposure to pollutants common in driving and industrial situations "may become less effective in coping effectively with unexpected events and more liable to perform routine tasks in an inefficient manner."

changing values and the loss of tradition

Change is also reflected in much less physical factors. Though abstract, cultural changes are even more profound in their impact upon our overall health because they directly affect both our attitudes toward health and our ways of responding to disease. We are influenced by— and must be alert to—new developments in social values, family life, and the code models offered to us.

Our lives are unquestionably easier (and potentially more fun-filled) than those of our ancestors. Life in the old days was relatively undiversified, and certainly more brutal. Yet problems were simpler, more direct, and in many ways more predictable than today's constant, cumulative annoyances. Today's events seem beyond the immediate control of the individual, an ironic development since technology was to have given us greater command of our lives. According to a poll taken by the Institute of Life Insurance, only 58 percent of the population in 1968 felt they had personal control over key areas of their lives. By 1976 that number had plummeted to 39 percent.

In less complicated times, people dealt with a small number of other people whose behavior they could predict reasonably well, and whose values and attitudes were easy to comprehend. The abstractions they had to deal with were associated with raw nature, or God. Intimately connected to these abstract forces through constantly reinforced religious and cultural traditions, individuals could accept, understand, and justify even tumultuous events that were out of their control.

For our ancestors, change was less incessant, and they had anchors to buffer its impact. Sources of solace and adjustment were built into cultural patterns, assuaging loss before it could become an ulcer or a coronary. As our connections with nature and human community have eroded, we have lost important psychological tools for adaptation. In an important *Fortune* article on stress in 1972, Walter McQuade described the phenomenon in this way:

> Modern societies have to a great extent lost the supports that helped people in earlier times endure toil, hardship, and suffering—religious faith, sustaining frameworks of tradition and custom, a sense of place in the social order, a sense of worth derived from the exercise of craftsmanship, and awareness that toil, hardship, and suffering were likewise endured by the other members of the same community and the same social class.

This is not to glamorize the simple life, which offered harsh, often brutal, challenges on the one hand and humdrum routine on the other, but to point out the unique nature of today's sources of illness.

"At the moment, I would say the most frequent causes of distress in man are psychological," says Dr. Hans Selye, the pioneer in stress research. "That is to say, lack of adaptability, not having a code of behavior. One reason for this is that the satisfaction of religious codes has diminished in importance for mankind. So has the idea of being loyal to your monarch or leader."

That the decline of spiritual values is largely responsible for our high incidence of stress disorders is agreed upon by many authorities. "Those who believe in a positive God and prayer are happier and healthier people and therefore ought to live longer," says Dr. Curt G. Batiste. "Believing there is a Father up there who will help you reduces stress and saves wear and tear on the heart."

Lest he be accused of evangelizing, Dr. Batiste, a psychiatrist, adds: "I don't believe in God myself, but I suspect it is easier for those who believe in God to get through difficult times than for those who don't."

We not only have severed ourselves from the simple society of our fathers, but we change our own with astonishing speed. Fads and fashions, a myriad of fluctuating ideas, philosophies, and world-views all shape and reshape our awareness more often in the course of a few months than was the case in decades, even centuries, for our ancestors.

We even shift locations with incredible frequency. Each year since 1948 one of every five Americans changed addresses. The average home owner stays in a single home for a mere seven years. Between March 1967 and March 1968, over 36 million Americans changed their place of residence. Alvin Toffler points out that the magnitude of such a shift, in terms of numbers, is as if the total combined populations of Cambodia, Ghana, Guatamala, Honduras, Iraq, Israel, Mongolia, Nicaragua, and Tunisia were to have picked up and relocated.

Moving corresponds to other changes. The average American switches jobs every three years, and that brings about a plethora of other changes—in habit, social ties, climate, and schooling. "All change involves loss of some kind," observes Dr. Alan McLean, area medical director at IBM. "Familiar faces, places, pleasures, ways of doing things, or organizational supports. Promotions, demotions, and transfers, however desired, are changes. Such losses are more severe than many persons recognize. Change is a threat to the ways people have developed to handle their dependency needs."

The Changing Family

Perhaps the greatest indication, and one of the most crushing symptoms, of the erosion of tradition is the transformation of family life. Referring to "an upheaval that is changing the canvas of American society" *New York Times* reporter Jon Nordheimer writes that "nowhere is the impact more intense, the confusion greater, than in the family, where stress sends repercussions throughout society, from the games children play, to education, courtship, and the labor market."

---

changes in family life

The following statistics chronicle the drastic changes in the structure of family life:

Nearly half of all marriages end in divorce.
An estimated 40 percent of the children born in this decade will spend at least part of their youth in homes with only one parent.
Households headed by women have doubled in the last generation and increased by a third in the last ten years.
A third of the women with children under age three work outside the home.
The percentage of people aged 20–34 who have never married has increased by 10 to 20 percent in the last sixteen years.
The number of unmarried couples living together has more than doubled since 1960.

The experts, predictably, are at odds about the interpretation of these trends. Some see them as an indication of a new, advanced civilization in which the family will take on new more appropriate forms. Others see it as a sign of the destruction of values that have sustained humankind throughout its history. They agree on one thing: we are not likely to return soon to the ways of the past. Even if the nuclear family is strengthened and men and women once again provide stable, lifelong homes for themselves and their children, social mobility and other factors will prevent the return of the extended family structure and the close-knit geographical community with roots and continuity.

Changing Roles for Men and Women

In less than a generation, the roles played by men and women have undergone greater change than they have in centuries of Western civilization. Perhaps for the first time in history there are no clear-cut, universally agreed-upon standards of action for the most basic human interactions. Says marriage counselor Michael Kelso, quoted in the *New York Times*:

> After a while you begin to sense that their real problem is that they feel lost, confused, and alienated because the roles of being a husband or a wife or a parent have changed so much from the days when they were kids. They no longer know what the standards and values of family life are today. They don't know what to tell their kids.

Eli Ginzberg, chairman of the National Commission for Manpower

Policy, calls the changing roles of men and women the "single most outstanding phenomenon of this century. It is a worldwide phenomenon, an integral part of a changing economy and a changing society. Its secondary and tertiary consequences are really unchartable."

---

women at work

Fully 48.9 percent of women over 16 are now in the labor market, including half of all mothers with school-age children. That represents 40.5 million women, a figure fast approaching the 57.2 million working males. Economists predict that the percentage will rise to 50 percent in the next ten years and that six women will enter the work force for every five men.

The changing participation of women in the extrafamilial activities of society has stirred controversy in academic and scientific circles. Biologists and social scientists are still trying to determine the degree to which social roles are genetically influenced. Increasing numbers of women taking professional positions in business have had an enormous impact on the corporate world, where men must deal with female bosses and peers for the first time, and where women executives find themselves in a pioneer role for which there are no precedents and no models to emulate.* That, in turn, has led to rebound effects on the home, where the sudden presence of two parents rushing off to catch the 7:32 has opened a Pandora's box of petty problems, all adding up to a difficult adjustment in home life. "Everybody's in favor of equal pay," said one researcher, "but nobody's in favor of doing the dishes."

—————— the changing nature of work ——————

At the turn of the century John Pierpont Morgan is reported to have complained that his organization was getting too big. "I don't even know everyone on my staff by first name," he protested.

By today's standards, Morgan's empire would be considered a small business. In 1911 the Supreme Court, leery of giant trust companies, split the "octopus" Standard Oil Company into 11 separate companies. Today, according to Peter Drucker, each of those 11 companies is "larger than the original Standard Oil Company ever was—in capital, in employees, in production. Yet only four of them rank among the major American, let alone the major international, oil companies today."

---

*The impact of the emerging managerial woman will be discussed further in a subsequent chapter.

The sustenance of virtually every civilization, and the institution around which the great majority of work was performed has always been agriculture. At the time of the American Revolution fully three-quarters of the nation worked on farms. Today, despite the fact that our agriculture industry feeds over 350 million people throughout the world, less than 6 percent work on farms, and many of those work for aggregates whose size rivals industrial firms.

Even late in the nineteenth century, most businesses were small, family-owned enterprises, with relatively few functions. Then, spurred by the opportunity for increased productivity, the activities of many enterprises became increasingly subsumed under the heading of a single company. The resulting large, multiunit corporation drastically transformed the way individuals work. Among other things, it required the creation of a new category of professional—the manager.

The Managerial Dimension

Decisions concerning hiring and firing, wages, hours, and working conditions were increasingly transferred from the hands of the foreman to the plant manager and ultimately to the desks of executives in a central office. More important, notes Alfred Chandler, author of *The Visible Hand,* the modern business managers "took over the functions of coordinating flows of goods through existing processes of production and distribution, and of allocating funds and personnel for future production and distribution." Previously this occurred through natural market mechanisms—Adam Smith's "invisible hand."

This has resulted in a major transformation in the world of work in a remarkably short period of time. Even relatively small businesses have a hierarchy of managers who make major decisions but do not own the enterprise that they represent. But many observers feel that the way executives have been trained to think reflects the economy of a different era. "Much basic economic theory," Chandler maintains, "is still grounded on the assumption that the processes of production and distribution are managed, or at least should be managed, by small traditional enterprises regulated by the invisible hand of the market."

The Changing Work Force

The same century that saw human enterprise shift radically from the fields to the cities saw America become the first nation in which more than half the labor force consisted of white-collar workers. We now work in huge groups that attempt to bring large numbers of diverse skills together under one coordinated enterprise, something that previous generations found hard to do even when the numbers of people and the range of skills were countable on one's fingers.

In addition, the overwhelming majority of individuals perform their services for rewards that are more abstract and more removed from their actual labor than did previous generations. Few people work at jobs that are directly linked to the end product—the merchandise, the food, or the consumer.

The Changing Structure of Business

Titles, job descriptions, responsibilities, departments, divisions now are created and dismantled at an alarming rate. Says management consultant D. R. Daniel, "One major restructuring every two years is probably a conservative estimate of the current rate of organizational change among the largest industrial corporations."

Rapid change is dramatized by the rise of project and task-force management, where teams of people are assembled to work on short-range projects and are disbanded as soon as the project is completed. A growing number of professionals are constantly on the move from company to university to foundation to government to another company. The old loyalty to the company is giving way to new loyalties— to one's profession or industry, rather than to one's organization.

Before we have adjusted to managerial capitalism, a whole array of new issues has arisen to demand still further adaptability from business. Increased government intervention, depletion of energy resources, demands for corporate accountability, the women's movement, and the widespread desire of employees for satisfaction beyond bread-winning, have all conspired to complicate still further the day-to-day world of work.

Decision Stress

Rational decisions depend upon the ability to predict the consequences of one's actions. Today, this requires processing extraordinary amounts of information at extreme speed. We must weigh a greater number of alternatives in much less time than our predecessors. Yet, experiments have shown that the greater the number of alternatives open to a person, the longer it takes to reach a decision and act upon it. As Henry Kissinger once said, "The absence of alternatives clears the mind marvelously."

Experiments have also revealed two basic principles that could explain the breakdowns suffered by executives who deal with "decision stress" day in and day out: humans have a limited capacity to receive, process, and remember information (just how limited is open to debate, as is the question of whether or not this capacity can be improved). Overloading the system can lead to a serious breakdown in performance.

In addition, we face what Daniel Yankelovich, president of the public-opinion polling firm of Yankelovich, Skelly, and White, calls a "qualitative difference in the decision-making process."

Yankelovich distinguishes between risk and uncertainty. In the former, you may know the variables that influence a situation, but not the amount of weight to give each one. In the case of uncertainty, you don't even know what the variables are. Too much uncertainty destroys the ability to maintain stability and control.

Executives are trained to measure and control risk factors. By virtue of that training, and probably by virtue of psychological makeup as well (managers tend to score high on tests that measure the need to influence and control), an executive's strongest trait is the ability to control and manage the variables with which he or she is confronted. This, claims Yankelovich, makes executives less tolerant of uncertainty.

Holistic Decision Making

Quantification; systematic, rational thinking; tight lines of control; rigorous priority setting—these have been the executive's tools, and they have worked remarkably well. They work best under conditions of normal risk, however, not under conditions of uncertainty. Today's world increasingly calls upon other skills, other traits, other faculties.

Confronted by an increasing rate of uncertainty, the executive is likely to experience growing anxiety. Falling back on his usual way of dealing with risk will not work. There is no analytic, computer-like way of dealing with the unknown. Only the intuitive faculties, which scientists are just beginning to understand, can cope effectively with uncertainty. Yankelovich, therefore, calls for "higher sensitivity, sounder judgement, greater openness to change and new experience, and a larger, broader focus on the whole rather than just detailed knowledge of specific subjects and methods."

Executives are dealing, then, with a world in transition. Predictability and control, important safeguards against disease-provoking stress, seem increasingly unattainable. Many observers feel that the democratization and debureaucratization of the classical hierarchy, and the increased freedom enjoyed by professionals are welcome signs of adaptation to changes taking place in society. Welcome or not, they bring new sets of pressures to which executives must adapt.

Work overload, too much responsibility with too little authority, difficult subordinates, conflicting job demands, role ambiguity—all frequently mentioned as sources of stress disorders—can probably be traced to the larger issue of rapid change. Under such novel conditions people are forced to behave quite differently, and the new ways of acting (whatever they may be) have not yet become a matter of routine. Some doubt that they ever will be. Perhaps the only thing we can count on is more change.

These new sources of stress contribute to a work environment that seems to be taking its toll:

According to studies done by Kahn et al. (reported in *Occupational Stress*, Charles C. Thomas, 1974) only one in six persons claims to be relatively free of stress, while 83 percent feel they are experiencing a great deal of stress as a result of their jobs.

According to the *New York Times*, a study of 800 executives over a three-year period showed a high correlation between anxiety and reported health problems on the one hand and job satisfaction and perceived job stress on the other; *no* correlation existed between anxiety levels and salary, number of hours worked, or commuting time.

---

major life changes and disease

Dr. Thomas Holmes and Dr. Richard Rahe, of the University of Washington School of Medicine, have studied the clinical effects of major life changes. Over some 20 years, Holmes and Rahe had representatives of diverse racial and ethnic backgrounds in the United States and abroad rank specific life changes according to their degree of impact on health. To their astonishment, there was virtually universal agreement.

As a result of copious interviews, Holmes and Rahe were able to assign a numerical value to each life event, ranking them in order of magnitude. Then they compared the life-change scores of some 5000 individuals with their respective medical histories. Those who had a high rating on the life-change index were more likely to contract illness following the events.

The "Schedule of Recent Events" has since been applied to a wide variety of groups, always confirming the notion that the higher the degree of life change within a given period of time, the greater the risk of subsequent illness, regardless of whether or not the change was perceived as desirable or undesirable.

It is interesting to note that, of the 36 events, only ten are decidedly negative (although five of those are in the top six), six are decidedly positive, and the rest, 20, are so worded that one can only call them neutral.

---

self-evaluation: compute your life change risk

Which of these changes occurred in your life this past year? Add up the point values of each event.

Event	Life-Change Units		
Death of a spouse	100	Son or daughter leaving	
Marital separation	65	home	29
Death of a close family		Trouble with in-laws	29
member	63	Outstanding personal	
Personal injury or illness	53	achievement	28
Marriage	50	Wife beginning or stopping	
Loss of job	47	work	29
Marital reconciliation	45	Revision of personal habits	24
Retirement	45	Trouble with business	
Change in health of a		superior	23
family member	44	Change in work hours	
Wife's pregnancy	40	or conditions	20
Sex difficulties	39	Change in residence	20
Gain of a new family		Change in schools	20
member	39	Change in recreation	19
Change in financial status	38	Change in social activities	18
Death of a close friend	37	Taking out a small	
Change to a different kind		mortgage on your home	17
of work	36	Change in sleeping habits	16
Increase or decrease in		Change in number of	
arguments with spouse	35	family get-togethers	15
Taking out a big mortgage		Change in eating habits	15
on home	31	Vacation	13
Foreclosure of mortgage		Minor violations of law	11
or loan	30		
Change in work responsibilities			

If your life-change units total 150–199 you stand a mild chance of incurring some form of illness in the next year. If the total is 200–299 LCUs you are a moderate risk. Over 300 points puts you in the group very likely to suffer serious physical or emotional illness.

A "Typical" Life-Change Score

Let us follow the life of a fictitious executive for one year. For purposes of illustration, we will protect him from the five biggest stressors and keep the year as positive as possible. Even so, the points pile up.

As a result of a notable personal achievement (28 LCUs), Mr. Henderson was promoted from division manager to the executive ranks. His move to the company's executive headquarters in the city carried with it a large raise (38 LCUs), as well as several other changes. Henderson's responsibilities increased considerably (29), and the nature of the work itself now required dealing with more "people problems" than he was used to (36).

Henderson acquired a new wardrobe that better fit his executive status. That, and the new routes he had to travel to downtown, represented a considerable change in habits (24). He had to wake up an hour earlier (16). In addition, his lunches were no longer casual; at least four of five were business lunches, with richer food than he was accustomed to (15). As a result of his new routine, Henderson was forced to give up his weekly tennis game, but he made up for it by taking up squash at a club in the city (19). Henderson enjoyed those changes and the new weekend social activities that opened up to him once he got to know his new colleagues (18). At first, he didn't even mind the longer hours that he had to put in (20).

When he realized that the new job was cutting into his time with the family (15), he decided to move to a more convenient location. He took out a mortgage on a fine home (31), and moved in without a moment's delay (20).

Henderson and his wife had been having trouble in recent years, but the new events seemed to bring back some of the old romance. They did not argue as much as they had been (35). No longer pressured by financial problems, Henderson's wife was able to stop working (29).

A few months after the family had settled into their new home, Henderson's daughter announced that she was getting married. He was losing a daughter, of course, (29) but gaining a son (39). The wedding plans were complicated and stirred up some old difficulties with Henderson's in-laws (29). Mrs. Henderson, exhausted by the tumult of the wedding, came down with an allergic reaction that required a brief hospitalization (44). It was nothing serious, but Henderson thought it was a good excuse to take a trip to the Bahamas (13).

In that altogether plausible sequence of events—most of which could only be interpreted as desirable—Henderson accumulated a whopping 527 life-change units, which puts him way up there on the danger list.

If you subtract some of the decidedly negative events—his wife's illness, the difficulties with the in-laws, the mortgage, and the longer hours—he is still way over the 300 mark. If, on the other hand, you add a personal illness, trouble with the boss, or a death, his score rockets to double the critical 300 mark.

Regulating Change

Does all this mean we should try not to change? Hardly. Change is the stuff of life. We couldn't avoid change if we wanted to, and none of us would.

What it might mean is that we should try to regulate the changes in our lives, most of which are under our control, and try to keep them from coming too quickly or too intensely. The values assigned to the Holmes-Rahe scale are, of course, averages. Your personal reactions may deviate from those figures. Keep alert to the impact of various life changes on you. Then try to manage your life so that the hardest-hitting changes come with some distance between them.

─────── what is the bottom line? ───────

We have a picture of modern men and women, called upon to adapt to a world that is qualitatively and quantitatively more different from our fathers' world than theirs was from Julius Caesar's. Family life is changing, social life is changing, the world of work is changing, all with astonishing speed. Our adaptive skills are being taxed on all levels —physically, psychologically, emotionally, spiritually. The resulting stress leads to a slew of biochemical upheavals that is probably responsible for most of our modern maladies.

"To survive," writes Alvin Toffler, "the individual must become infinitely more adaptable and capable than ever before. He must search out totally new ways to anchor himself, for all the old roots—religion, nation, community, family, or profession—are now shaking under the hurricane impact of accelerative thrust."

the current score

It all boils down to this:

Coronary disease has increased 500 percent in the last 50 years.
An estimated 30 million Americans have some form of major heart or blood-vessel disease.
An estimated one million have heart attacks each year.

> *Of those, 650,000—including 200,000 between ages 45 and 65—die.*
> *Approximately one of every five men will have a coronary attack before age 60.*
> *For every death due to industrial accidents, there are 50 for cardiovascular disease.*
> *About 25 million Americans have hypertension (high blood pressure).*
> *Approximately 60,000 die each year of hypertension, not counting those whose high blood pressure precipitates a heart attack or stroke.*
> *An estimated eight million Americans have ulcers.*
> *10,000 die each year of hemorrhages or abdominal perforations that result from peptic ulcers.*
> *Approximately one in every eight persons suffers with migraine headaches at some time.*
> *12 million Americans are said to be alcoholics.*
> *Approximately ten million are diabetics.*
> *Americans consume 16,000 tons of aspirin each year, at an expenditure of approximately 500 million dollars.*
> *More than 230 million prescriptions are filled each year, including five billion doses of tranquilizers, three billion doses of amphetamines, and five billion doses of barbiturates.*
> *Ten percent of American males now aged 45 will not make it to 55.*

Where to Invest for Health

It sounds grim. But we humans have an outstanding adaptive trait that has served us well—creative intelligence. By all indications, this period of unsurpassed challenge—this so-called Age of Stress—is being weathered and conquered thanks to the American genius for recognizing the useful and inventing the impossible. Experts from all fields of human endeavor have responded to the problem of stress with a cornucopia of procedures that, if used properly, promises to reverse the disease-strewn path we have been on.

There are already some indications that a healthy upswing is underway. In the winter of 1978, Dr. Robert I. Levy, director of the National Heart, Lung, and Blood Institute, announced that there has been a decline in the death rate from cardiovascular disease. In 1976, the total number of deaths from heart and blood-vessel disorders dropped below one million for the first time since 1967. "We seem to have turned the corner in the epidemic of heart disease," said Dr. Levy.

What is responsible for the improvement? Most experts feel that the life-style changes extolled by physicians for two decades have finally been adopted by enough people to have made an impact. Total consumption of saturated fats and cholesterol has dropped; tobacco consumption has declined by 24 percent since 1964; an estimated 50 percent of those with high blood pressure are now being adequately treated, as opposed to only 12 percent in 1970; exercise has skyrocketed in popularity, as have various forms of relaxation.

Authorities believe that the new statistics vindicate their preventive measures and suggest that cardiovascular disease can be overcome. But, despite the improvement, there is still a long way to go. The American rate of heart disease is still one of the world's highest. "A broad, sustained societal effort must be mounted to continue and expand these efforts," says Dr. Jeremiah B. Stamler, chief of preventive medicine at Northwestern University Medical School.

Our habits, our priorities, and our life-styles have all been called into question. Newer, healthier ways of living are being advocated by health experts. These will be discussed in the second part of this book, but first we must have a clear understanding of stress so that we may hope to tame it. To do this, we must define it (chapter two), learn to recognize its effects (chapter three), minimize these effects (chapter four), and, most importantly, strive holistically to prevent them through an informed program of coordinated health practices tailored to our own individual needs (chapters five through nine).

what is stress and what does it do?

---

self-evaluation: a stress journal

To identify stress factors that you encounter regularly, keep a daily log, indicating each of your activities, its duration, and the degree of positive or negative stress it seems to carry. We recommend keeping the log for at least two weeks. Along with the information in this chapter, it will help you identify the stress response when it occurs. You will then be able to correct situations that cause too much stress.

Assign one of the following scores to each activity:

1. pleasant, enjoyable, and relaxing
2. pleasant but taxing (perhaps hurried)
3. necessary (neither pleasant nor unpleasant) but taxing
4. unpleasant, hurried, or tension producing
5. very unpleasant, pressured, and tension producing

Here is an example of a morning's log:

Activity	From–To	Stress Score
Shower and breakfast	7:00–7:45	2
Drive to work	7:45–8:30	3
Read mail	8:30–9:00	2
Meeting with staff	9:00–10:30	4
Dictate letters	10:30–11:15	2

If you find many days with 1 1/2 or more hours spent in categories 4 and 5, you should consider how to alter your routine, whether it means scheduling fewer appointments, delegating more responsibility, taking the train instead of driving, having fewer business lunches, or whatever. Aim for low point scores.

the definition of stress

Like many scientific terms that find their way into the popular lexicon, stress has taken on a variety of meanings. "The word is getting beaten to death," bemoans Dr. Sidney Lecker, director of the StressControl Center, an affiliate of Executive Health Examiners. "Everybody is using it in so many different ways that stress has totally lost its meaning. Stress is a very specific biological concept that relates to disease and disease prevention."

Nonetheless, Lecker and most medical experts applaud the growing awareness of stress, even if it means living with a muddled popular usage. "I'm happy it caught on," he concedes. "Nothing has ever gotten anybody interested in prevention before."

The acknowledged father of stress research, and the man most responsible for bringing the concept to the public's attention, is Dr. Hans Selye, a Vienna-born endocrinologist associated with the University of Montreal.

"It is important that people understand what they are talking about when they speak about stress," he says. "Whenever anyone experiences something unpleasant, for lack of a better word they say they are under stress."

In his classic book, *The Stress of Life,* Selye lists several incorrect notions of what stress is. Among them:

Stress is not nervous tension. This is the most popular use of the word,
as in "I'm feeling terribly stressed with this meeting coming up."
Stress is not the discharge of hormones from the adrenal glands. The

*common association of adrenalin with stress is not totally false, but
the two are only indirectly related, as we shall see.*

*Stress is not simply the influence of some negative occurence. Stress
can be caused by quite ordinary, and even positive, events ("a game
of tennis or even a passionate kiss," writes Selye).*

*Stress is not an entirely bad event. We all need a certain amount of
stimulation in life and most people can thrive on some forms of
stress.*

*Stress does not cause the body's alarm reaction. This is the most com-
mon misuse of the word. What causes the stress reaction is the
stressor.*

These nondefinitions seem to eliminate just about everything.
What, then, is stress? To paraphrase Selye, it is a *state,* manifested by
a specific syndrome of biological events. Very specific changes occur in
the biological system, but these changes are caused by such a wide
variety of agents that, strictly speaking, we must call stress *nonspecifi-
cally induced.* But the key to understanding the nature of this overall
biological impact lies in the fact that *some* stress response, however
slight, will result from *any* stimulus. *Stress* is the nonspecific response
of the body to any demand made upon it. In more colloquial terms, we
might define stress as the rate of wear and tear caused by life.

the general adaptation syndrome

In its broadest sense, stress is some taxation of the body's resources in
order to respond to some environmental circumstance. Clinically, the
study of stress is based upon the more extreme instances of this response. In essence, the stress response is a mobilization of the body's
defenses, an ancient biochemical survival mechanism that was per-
fected during the evolutionary process, allowing human beings to
adapt to hostile or threatening events.

In 1936, Dr. Selye defined what he called the "general adaptation
syndrome," recognized as a major breakthrough in biological research.
It consists of three stages: alarm, resistance, and exhaustion.

1. THE ALARM REACTION When a stressor is recognized, the brain
sends forth a biochemical messenger to the pituitary gland, which
secretes adrenocorticotrophic hormone (ACTH). ACTH causes the adrenal glands to secrete corticoids such as adrenalin. This results in a
general call-to-arms to all the body's systems.

2. THE RESISTANCE STAGE Once the immediate threat dissipates,
or is overcome, the body tries to return to equilibrium. In many ways
this stage is the opposite of the alarm stage, whose characteristic physi-

ology fades and disappears as the organism adapts to the derangement caused by the stressor.

3. THE EXHAUSTION STAGE If the stressor continues, the acquired adaptation is eventually lost, and the new stage is entered. The symptoms of the initial alarm reaction return. If the stress is unduly prolonged, the wear and tear incurred will result in damage to a local area or death to the organism as a whole.

---

three stages of the general adaptation syndrome

Stage 1:	Alarm	Integrated call-to-arms. Intense readiness and mobilization of biochemical resources.
Stage 2:	Resistance	Vital resources applied to enable body to resist and adapt to the stressor.
Stage 3:	Exhaustion	Reversal to alarm stage in face of prolonged stress. Results in wear and tear, or death.

---

anatomy of the "fight-or-flight" response

Imagine, if you will, a primitive hunter, squatting in the comfort of his cave, picking his teeth with a bone. Suddenly, in the light cast by his fire, he glimpses the shadow of a tiger. His body undergoes a torrent of changes through the complex transmissions of the sympathetic and parasympathetic nervous systems.

---

the alarm reaction for fight-or-flight

stored sugar and fats pour into the bloodstream to provide fuel for quick energy

the breath rate shoots up, providing more oxygen

red blood cells flood the bloodstream, carrying more oxygen to the muscles of the limbs and the brain

the heart speeds up and blood pressure soars, insuring sufficient blood supply to needed areas

blood-clotting mechanisms are activated to protect against injury

muscles tense in preparation for strenuous action

digestion ceases, so blood may be diverted to muscles and brain

perspiration and saliva increase

triggered by the pituitary gland, the endocrine system steps up hormone production

bowel and bladder muscles loosen
adrenalin pours into the system, as do the hormones epinephrin and
norepinephrin
the pupils dilate, allowing more light to enter
all senses are heightened

It is an elegant display of innate intelligence. The entire response is unimaginably complex, and yet it is choreographed with perfect precision in a flash, under the control of the hypothalamus, a tiny bundle of nerve cells in the brain, about the size of a thimble.

This so-called fight-or-flight response has been a vital survival mechanism, physiologists believe. It is still with us. However, it may be inadequate—even destructive—in the face of the stressors that are typical of modern life.

One of your managers makes a critical mistake; the president says he is thinking of moving your division to Afghanistan; your spouse hands you a bill; a car cuts you off at an intersection. In each of those instances—and dozens more each day—your body might react in the same way the caveman reacted upon spotting the tiger. The difference is you can't clout your manager, nor do you take off after the offending car. In fact, rarely in these modern situations is there any real fight or flight. But biochemically you are prepared for just that, a good deal of the time.

Because the fight-or-flight response gets relentlessly turned on without being used for its "intended" purpose, it can itself become a major source of distress. As Walter McQuade put it. "In broad terms, man the victorious predator now preys upon himself."

Under threatening conditions, the response *is* of course desirable. But when fired too often or for too long, the body may remain in a state of permanent mobilization. The result is, at best, chronic tension. Worse, the hormones secreted in such abundance can ultimately lead to damage in vital organs or to the nervous system itself, resulting in physical and psychological disorders.

Premature aging and early death are other likely consequences of excessive wear and tear. Dr. Selye believes that each of us, in effect, has an inherited supply of "adaptation energy," which, like oil deposits are gone once they are burned up. But when the supply of adaptation energy is depleted, says Selye, so too is life, since no way has yet been discovered to replenish the fund.

Selye's theory has its dissenters, who are not convinced that any such finite supply of adaptation energy exists, or, if it does, that it can't be replenished. Everyone agrees on the basic point, however. In Selye's words, "Stress becomes dangerous when it is unduly prolonged, comes too often, or concentrates on one particular organ of the body."

Just what these consequences are will be discussed in chapters three and four.

─────────────────────────── stress vs. stimulation ───────────

Scientists are quick to point out that stress is a distinct physiological state. *Not all stress is unpleasant.* In colloquial usage, of course, stress always has a pejorative connotation, but, as Dr. Selye puts it, "in common parlance, when we say someone is 'under stress,' we actually mean under excessive stress, or distress. . . ."

Selye believes that "stress is the spice of life," and that the absence of stress is death.* To be alive means to respond to stimulation from the environment. By responding to the challenges of the environment we experience the joy and exhilaration of achievement; through such adaptive achievement we grow. "There is such a thing as pleasant stress," explains Selye, "as in the case of the Olympic winner at the moment of his glory, or a conductor as his orchestra performs particularly well. They are just radiating excitement, and they are secreting all the stress hormones exactly the same as if they were dejected or had just heard of a death in the family."

Thus, a vulnerable individual is as likely to keel over upon hearing he won a lottery as is the tycoon who discovers he has lost his fortune. The person who innocently enters a room to the joyous shout of "Surprise!" is just as shaken, physiologically, as the one who hears "Stick 'em up!" The groom who paces the floor in anticipation of his wedding may suffer the same biochemical derangements as the one who suspects his sweetheart of dating another man. "It is immaterial whether the agent or situation we face is pleasant or unpleasant," writes Dr. Selye. "All that counts is the intensity of the demand for readjustment of adaptation."

There is ample evidence to support the notion that we need, indeed thrive on, a certain amount of stimulation. Toffler points out that experiments "point unequivocally to the existence of what might be called an 'adaptive range' below which and above which the individual's ability to cope simply falls apart."

Therefore, the answer to work stress is not simply more leisure time. Attitude surveys show that the overwhelming majority of individuals would choose to continue working even if they suddenly inherited enough money to be independently wealthy. The current

─────────

*Selye has coined the words "eustress" and "distress" to distinguish between positive and destructive forms of stress. These are key distinctions. To avoid confusion, however, we have chosen not to use technical terminology in this book, making the distinction with more colloquial language.

controversy over forced retirement supports the theory of positive stress. As Benjamin Franklin put it, "There is nothing wrong with retirement as long as one doesn't allow it to interfere with one's work."

Such seemingly harmless circumstances as rigid routine work are no less stressful even though they lack noxious infringement from outside sources. In fact, monotony can produce many of the same physiological symptoms as overwork—what psychiatrist Robert Seidenberg calls the "trauma of eventlessness." Suburban housewives, for example, whose lives are stable and secure, but relatively devoid of challenges or change, dread their situation as much as their husbands or working friends might dread a hectic day at the office.

Upper Echelon Stress

This might help explain a curious phenomenon that once bewildered experts. The common assumption is that executives at the top—those who determine policy and bear the heavier burden of responsibility—are those most prone to stress disease. Yet, a study of 1540 bank officers found that people with too *few* job-related stressors had as high an incidence of disorders as those with an abundance of stressors. "In other words," concludes Kathy Slobogin of the *New York Times*, "a worker tucked away in some peaceful department and given nothing to do is just as likely to drop dead of a heart attack as the highly pressured executive with too much to do."

A Metropolitan Life Insurance Company study kept track of the three top executives at Fortune 500 companies over a sixteen-year period. It was discovered that the mortality rate of men at the top was only 63 percent that of the rest of the white male population. In 1968, a study of 270,000 male employees at a major corporation showed that the rate of coronary disease was *lower* with each step up the occupational ladder.

There are several possible explanations, each of which carries some validity and contributes something to our understanding of the complexities of stress. The satisfaction of success serves as a restorative for added pressure ("resting at the peak is easier than making the climb," said one writer). It could also be that the middle rungs, where one is caught between policymaking decisions and execution, are inherently more stressful because of ambiguity and relative powerlessness. Furthermore, perhaps some people are constitutionally more resilient to certain kinds of stressors, a view that seems to have considerable validity in the business world—presumably the ones who make it to the top do so precisely because they are tough enough to come through the battle unscathed. "I don't get ulcers," said one real-estate tycoon. "I give them."

——————————————————————— **what makes
a stressor stressful?** ———

Individual Differences

The Chinese word for crisis is a combination of the symbols for two other words: danger and opportunity. Whether a given situation is a threat or a challenge is, of course, largely a matter of individual perception. So is the difference between sufficient stimulation and stress overload. "You can't make a race horse out of a turtle," says Dr. Selye. "But the reverse is also true. If you are the race-horse type, as most efficient business executives and politicians are, you have the urge to do many things and to express yourself. If you are told not to do anything, you are under terrible distress."

As for the turtles: "I respect the fellow who wants to be a beachcomber. What I condemn is the person born to be a beachcomber who forces himself to be an executive, even though he's not made for it and suffers as a result."

We all know people who can't stand cold, and others who amaze us by walking around barely covered up. Some people can drink all night and retain their wits, while others get looped with a sip of wine. And we've seen those who can run all day without getting winded, while others gasp for air if they run to catch a train. Just as there is wide variation in individual reactions to such physical stressors, there is equally wide variation to psychological and emotional stressors.

There is evidence to support the notion that those who find it difficult to adapt to challenging events are more vulnerable to illness in general. Says Dr. Harold Wolff, of Cornell University's Medical College: "Man's attempts to adapt to life situations which do not fulfill his needs, which frustrate his aspirations, or which place heavy conflicting demands upon him are very often associated with an increased susceptibility to all forms of illness."

Just what may account for all these individual differences has not yet been determined. A multitude of factors is involved—including differences in biochemistry, physical strength, psychological and emotional makeup, values, attitudes, habits, social setting, and others.

Since stress comes in all varieties, not just physical, a person's emotional and psychological strength goes a long way in determining resistance and vulnerability. This should be self-evident. Some people break down in the face of adversity, while others take it well, or are even spurred to heights of achievement. To say, therefore, that stress causes such psychological illnesses as depression or anxiety is to express only one side of the coin. It might be just as accurate to say that depression or anxiety *cause* stress.

In other words, stress works in a vicious cycle, a point that is often underplayed because it blurs the facile identification of causes and effects. Excessive stress leads to physical and psychological weaknesses of varying intensities. The person so afflicted does not function at full capacity. As a result, he or she is more vulnerable to future stress.

The stressed nervous system becomes less and less capable of withstanding the impact of stressors; immunity and resistance diminish; overload comes more quickly. In addition, individuals who have incurred wear and tear tend to encounter more stressful situations, since their efficiency of behavior is concomitantly impaired. Psychological weaknesses will lead to mistakes, poor interaction with family or coworkers, lack of confidence, and other sources of distress.

The cycle becomes a spiral as time goes on, and each successive encounter with stressors further weakens the individual. But, while such a pattern sounds bleak, leading ultimately to severe disorders, it can also be reversed. With the health procedures now available, already-existing disorders can be overcome, and simultaneously "immunity" to future stress overload can be heightened. Coping powers can be achieved through both physical and psychological skills, turning stressors into opportunities for growth. In this manner the satisfactions and rewards of hard work need not be sacrificed to obtain health and peace of mind. One can have success without distress.

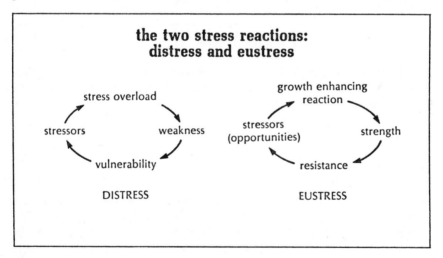

Control

Studies on humans indicate that lack of control is a key stress factor. A group of scientists attached pulse counters to the wrists of executives, who were to keep track of their activities all day. Among the situations that elicited the highest escalations of pulse was the simple act of driving to work. Why should that be so? The conclusion was that commuting, with its accompanying traffic jams and cars to dodge, represented a situation in which the person lacked control.

---

the need for control

In a classic study, monkeys were placed in an isolation booth and exposed to periodic flashing lights, increases in temperature, and electric shocks. Given a lever that shut off the stressor, the monkeys began to pump it constantly, even when the stressor was not on.

After a few weeks, the lever was moved; the monkeys could see it but they could not reach it. The stressors were also removed. Yet, despite their newly acquired freedom from harassment, the monkeys tried desperately to get their hands on the lever. Failing, twelve of the thirteen developed neurotic and psychosomatic symptoms; two got asthma; two developed duodenal ulcers and died; five had gastrointestinal disturbances and sores. The neurotic symptoms included apathy, suspension of grooming habits, catching imaginary flies, increased masturbatory behavior, and pulling out their own fur.

Two of the monkeys were allowed to operate the levers again. They made a dramatic recover. Why? Probably they felt they were in control.

In a similar study, scientists measured certain stress-related hormones in Swedish commuters. Those who boarded the train at the first stop, 79 minutes from Stockholm, were compared with those who boarded midway, 43 minutes from the destination. Both groups agreed that the ride seemed to become increasingly stressful as they approached Stockholm. But those who boarded earlier actually secreted *less* of the stress hormone.

Again, the key variable was felt to be control. Those who boarded at the first stop had greater freedom of choice. They could choose their own seat and find room for their coats on the luggage racks. They could sit next to whomever they wished. The group who boarded the train at the midway point had to scramble for seats, separate from their friends, and otherwise adapt to a situation over which they had little control.

In still another experiment, subjects were given concentrative tasks to perform while disturbances were going on in the background. Those who were told they could stop the disturbances any time they wanted to did significantly better than the others, *even though they did not bother to exercise the right.*

Such studies indicate a possible connection between job-related problems such as absenteeism, turnovers, dissatisfaction, and inefficiency and the simple feeling of having no control.

Predictability

Your expectations, your knowledge, and your anticipation of an event will each have a bearing on its impact. At New York's Rockefeller University two groups of rats were given electric shocks of equal intensity and frequency. However, one group heard a beeping tone exactly ten seconds before each shock, while the other heard the beeps at random, unpredictable intervals, unrelated to the timing of the shocks. Both groups developed ulcers, as expected. But the group with the unreliable forewarning had six times more.

Apparently, however, *over*anticipation can amplify stress, as in the case of a student worrying about a coming exam, or an executive approaching a conference with trepidation. Typically, stomachaches, rashes, and other symptoms of anxiety appear long before the actual event. It thus becomes a matter of intelligent anticipation and realistic predictability. Knowing a shock is coming can be just as distressing as having it come unannounced, if you don't know exactly when to expect it, or what it will entail.

Yale University psychiatrist Irving Janus reports that patients who —because they are ill-informed—are calm, unbothered, and unconcerned prior to surgery suffer the most afterward. Their jaunty attitudes turn to resentment, anxiety, depression, belligerence, anger, and grouchiness when suddenly confronted with the unexpected realities of postoperative discomfort.

On the other hand, those who are excessively intimidated and enter surgery jittery or even tearful are almost as bad afterward. Their fear continues to haunt them and they need constant reassurance.

According to Dr. Janus's research, those with a "moderate degree of anticipatory fear" adjust best. They ask for the facts and they rehearse their discomforts mentally in advance. They are psychologically inoculated against stress.

Individual Perception

An important study, with several interesting implications for businessmen, was done by Dr. Harold Wolff and Dr. Lawrence E. Hinkle. They gathered data over a long period of time on a large group of telephone company workers, and found significant differences between operators who were chronically ill and those who were in good health.

The former had backgrounds, aspirations, and interests that were incompatible with their positions. They tended to come from well-educated homes with professional parents, and saw their own work as confining, boring, and beneath them.

By contrast, the healthy group tended to come from lower middle-class backgrounds. They accepted their lot in life without questioning, they had a clear awareness of their own limitations, and were generally content. The "job-personality fit" was a good one.

In a very real sense, most events are neutral—they are what we make them. Promotions are a good example. To the man who desires and expects one, being overlooked can be awfully distressing. But not to the man who hadn't given promotion a second thought. Conversely, a promotion will be taken in stride by the former individual, whereas the latter may suffer great anxiety upon being offered a better position. One person's crisis is another's joy.

Intense Responsibility

Air traffic control is said to be one of the most hazardous jobs in the world. Only 2 of the 94 controllers and trainees at Chicago's O'Hare Airport, which reporter David Martindale calls "a ticket to hell," have worked there more than ten years. Nearly two-thirds of them have ulcers or show symptoms of ulcers. Since 1970, more than 35 controllers have been permanently removed from O'Hare for medical reasons; many of them are now in psychiatric care. High blood pressure is four times more prevalent than among pilots, whose *own* lives are in greater danger.

Other occupations require split-second decisions and the simultaneous evaluation of many complex factors. Yet they do not elicit quite the same level of stress disorders as air traffic control. Why? Because, say the experts, the controller's every decision affects thousands of other peoples' lives.

It can be argued, of course, that responsibility for other individuals is not the most significant factor at work in these statistics. It may have much to do with the type of personality that chooses the life of a doctor, or with working conditions, long irregular hours, exposure to illness, and other factors. Nevertheless, many experts feel the sheer weight of other people's safety and health is a key variable.

---

stress of responsibility

Physicians, who often have direct responsibility for many lives, are one of the most vulnerable professional groups.

One-fourth of deaths among physicians between ages 25 and 44 are suicides (only 8.5 percent of deaths among white male non-physicians in that age group are suicides).
The suicide rate of women physicians is three times higher than for women in the general population.
Physicians have the highest alcoholism rate among all professionals.
Physicians' suicide rate is 33 per 10,000 (psychiatrists are 59 in 10,000).
Narcotic addiction among physicians may be 30 to 100 times that of the general population.

Executives can readily identify with that. "Dollars, stockholder's dividends, market changes, all those are just numbers," said one vice-president at a large manufacturing company. "They bother me, sure, But the decisions that eat away at my gut are the ones that involve people. If I have to lay off the father of a family, or deny a transfer to someone, I'm a wreck for days."

—————————————————————————— **summary** ——————

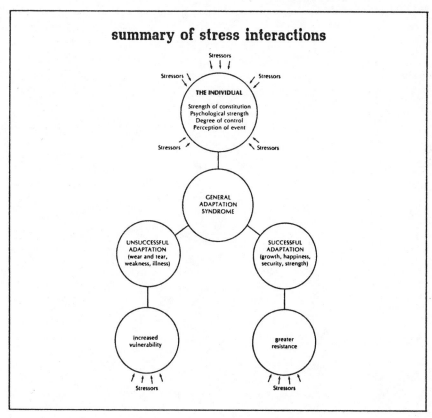

summary of stress interactions

Stressors
Stressors
Stressors

THE INDIVIDUAL
Strength of constitution
Psychological strength
Degree of control
Perception of event

Stressors
Stressors

GENERAL ADAPTATION SYNDROME

UNSUCCESSFUL ADAPTATION (wear and tear, weakness, illness)

SUCCESSFUL ADAPTATION (growth, happiness, security, strength)

increased vulnerability

greater resistance

Stressors

Stressors

Anything we respond to can be a stressor, and often we are not even aware of our response. While obviously dangerous or demanding situations maybe almost universally stress producing, every individual has different limits and vulnerabilities. More importantly, every one of us has a particular, unique blend of strengths and talents that can be either stimulated or paralyzed by stress that goes unchecked.

Ideally, this book would focus exclusively on preventing stress from obstructing health, but our civilization is only beginning to come to terms with the all-pervading nature of the problem. For this reason, we are all beginning our development of broad health programs somewhere in the middle of things—between intervention and prevention. Since the accumulation of stress can be extraordinarily subtle—until something ceases to work properly—early detection of both disease and stress disorders is a top priority in any approach to health.

The next chapter will survey the major areas of health that business people must come to understand, both for their own safety and the effectiveness of their employees and associates. Chapter four will then review what you can do to optimize detection if important disorders, and what medical science has to say about treating common stress-related problems.

the signs and symptoms of stress disorders

Many people assume that the absence of obvious tension implies they are relaxed. But a person can still have both the mental anxiety and the physical symptoms of prolonged, unabated stress without any noticeable discomfort. For these people, stress is so unremitting that they do not even recognize it any more; this lack of sensitivity can be dangerous in the long run.... When we ignore the signs of stress, we are training ourselves to take on a greater load of stress, rather than seeking means to alleviate it.   —Ken Pelletier, psychologist

self-evaluation

The following checklist is reprinted with permission of Don Isbell and Sally Nelson who direct a stress management program at Kaiser-Permanente in Southern California. The list will help you identify the particular ways in which stress manifests in your life. Some bodily systems are more reactive in one person than another. Too many C or F responses might indicate an organic illness is on the way.

Stress Symptom Checklist

Presented below are common problems which may be stress related. Please mark the frequency with which you have experienced each of these problems during the past two (2) months. Use the following symbols in responding on the checklist:

X - haven't had this problem at all
C - constant or nearly constant occurrence
F - frequently
O - occasionally

1. Tension headaches _____
2. Sleep-onset insomnia _____
3. Fatigue _____
4. Overeating _____
5. Constipation _____
6. Lower back pain _____
7. Allergy problems _____
8. Feelings of nervousness _____
9. Nightmares _____
10. High blood pressure _____
11. Hives _____
12. Alcohol/nonprescription drug consumption _____
13. Low-grade infections _____
14. Stomach indigestion _____
15. Hyperventilation _____
16. Worrisome thoughts _____
17. Dermatitis _____
18. Menstrual distress _____
19. Nausea or vomiting _____
20. Irritability _____
21. Migraine headaches _____
22. Early morning awakening _____
23. Loss of appetite _____
24. Diarrhea _____
25. Aching neck and shoulder muscles _____
26. Asthma attack _____
27. Colitis attack _____
28. Periods of depression _____
29. Arthritis _____
30. Common flu or cold _____
31. Minor accidents _____
32. Prescription drug use _____
33. Peptic ulcer _____
34. Cold hands or feet _____
35. Heart palpitations _____
36. Sexual problems _____
37. Angry feelings _____
38. Other _____

the warning signs

An important step in the prevention of stress disorders is to learn to identify those moments when you are undergoing the stress response. It is best to look for physiological signs, since the mental and emotional events that take place simulanteously can be deceptive. As we stated earlier, stress can be incurred even during happy events. Furthermore, in situations of excessive stress, you are likely to be so overshadowed by the emotions that your judgement and control will be impeded.

As we have seen, no two people react in exactly the same way to a stressful occurrence. One might become withdrawn and depressed, while another might become hyperactive, compulsive, or abnormally gregarious. One loses his appetite, while another becomes gluttonous;

one sleeps incessantly, another gets insomnia. Nonetheless, there are certain common indications of long-term wear and tear, and of present stress.

---

signs of fight-or-flight

The most telling indications that the fight-or-flight response is turned on *right now* are these:

rapid pulse
increased perspiration
pounding heart
tightened stomach
tensing of muscles in arms and legs
shortness of breath
gritting of teeth
clenching of the jaw
inability to sit still
racing thoughts
excessively gripping emotions

Prevention

Experts agree that an important preventive measure is to reverse the stress response when it is fired off inappropriately. This requires becoming sensitive to the particular ways you react to stress, and the situations that elicit the response (your stress journal will help). Learn to employ relaxation methods at those times. Abdominal breathing or muscle relaxation are the most commonly recommended devices; once mastered, they can be used inconspicuously, and without interfering with your activity. They are described in Chapter 8.

"The principle underlying physical stress control is that it is impossible for anyone to exist in two contradictory states simultaneously," writes Dr. Sidney Lecker, director of New York's Stress Control Center. "It is impossible to be stressed and physically relaxed at the same time. If you know how to find the state of physical relaxation and how to sustain it, you will be better able to prevent the occurence of physical stress overload and will be able to control excessive tension once it has occurred."

Underload vs. Overload

Executives should take note of the differences between stress overload and the strain of too little stimulation. They and their associates are, at times, subjected to either form of stress and should learn to respond appropriately to either situation.

Dr. Rosalind Forbes, director of the Denver-based Forbes Associates, is a psychologist who has specialized in corporate stress for over seven years. The following diagram depicts her concept of the continuum of underload—overload.

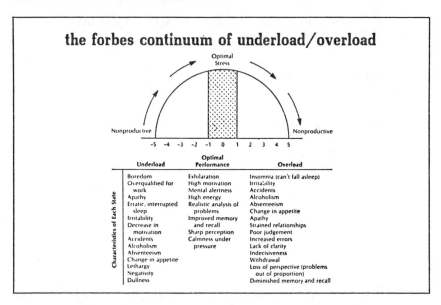

the forbes continuum of underload/overload

	Underload	Optimal Performance	Overload
Characteristics of Each State	Boredom	Exhilaration	Insomnia (can't fall asleep)
	Overqualified for work	High motivation	Irritability
	Apathy	Mental alertness	Accidents
	Erratic, interrupted sleep	High energy	Alcoholism
	Irritability	Realistic analysis of problems	Absenteeism
	Decrease in motivation	Improved memory and recall	Change in appetite
	Accidents	Sharp perception	Apathy
	Alcoholism	Calmness under pressure	Strained relationships
	Absenteeism		Poor judgement
	Change in appetite		Increased errors
	Lethargy		Lack of clarity
	Negativity		Indecisiveness
	Dullness		Withdrawal
			Loss of perspective (problems out of proportion)
			Diminished memory and recall

Both ends of the spectrum represent departures from optimal performance, and are precursors of physical and mental breakdowns. Everyone should find his or her "optimal stress level" for well-balanced stimulation, responsibility, and challenge.

don't ignore the warning signs

A great many executives make light of the warning signs of illness, perhaps subconsciously viewing them as a threat to their esteem or their careers. They may joke, play down the reliability of a doctor's diagnosis, or otherwise try to convince themselves and their associates that they are invulnerable. "I had mild chest pains for a year," admitted a Columbus, Ohio, businessman. "It was angina [chest pains that are a precursor of heart attacks], but I insisted that it was indigestion and kept munching antacid tablets." He ended up with cardiac arrest.

Psychological Clues

Serious disorders are often preceded by changes in personality or behavior. Excessive stress will elicit these signs while simultaneously eating away at the body's vital systems. When you find yourself thinking, "George had better take it easy or he'll get a heart attack," or, "If Tom doesn't stop worrying, he'll give himself an ulcer," take your observation seriously.

self-evaluation: psychological warnings

Watch out for changes like these:

Working late, or more obsessively than usual, or harder than seems appropriate to the situation. Sleeping at the office frequently is an important sign.

Difficulty making decisions, large and small, that the person would normally make easily.

Making the safe choices, not the best ones.

Excessive daydreaming or fantasizing; always wishing he or she were elsewhere.

Sexual or romantic indiscretions.

Sudden increase in drinking or smoking habits.

Use of antidepressants, tranquilizers, or mind-altering drugs.

Vague, disconnected speech or writing.

Excessive worrying, especially over relative trivia (or, extreme casualness and unconcern in the face of real problems).

Constant repetition of the same subject at meetings, especially if the point is not particularly important.

Inappropriate anger, hostility, or outbursts of temper.

Excessive or irrational mistrust of associates.

Constant harping on personal failures or shortcomings.

Constant reference to death or suicide.

Hypochondria.

Insomnia (either difficulty falling asleep or frequent awakenings).

Missing appointments or deadlines.

Confusing or forgetting dates, places, times, or other details.

Sudden propensity for mistakes.

Feeling worthless, inadequate, rejected, insecure (these are often hard to recognize, but might be evident between the lines).

Prolonged periods of brooding.

Difficulty getting along with other people.

Sudden reversals of usual behavior:

    an efficient worker becoming careless
    a casual worker becoming obsessively compulsive
    lavish spending by a normally frugal person
    excessive stinginess in a normally generous person
    aloofness in a normally friendly person
    extreme gregariousness in a normally shy person
    tendency to work alone by a "team player"
    sudden need to always be with others by an "independent type"

> *cheating, dishonesty, or breaches of ethics by a normally upright*
> *person*
> *shirking responsibilities usually accepted happily*

Naturally, most people display some of these symptoms some of the time. When they occur in patterns, if one or two persist, or if they occur with undisguised intensity, it is time to pay serious attention to the person's condition. He or she may be headed for a mental breakdown or a serious ailment, which in most cases can be averted if the behavioral warning signs are heeded.

The signs are often too subtle to notice, particularly if the observer and observed are the same person. Also, mental or behavioral problems usually manifest as exaggerations of the person's usual characteristics. "Mental illness," states Dr. Ralph Hirschowitz of Harvard, "is the extreme of a tendency already present in the individual. A mistrustful person could develop paranoia, while an enthusiastic, energetic type might become hypermanic."

An annual physical examination might reveal mental problems about to reach the boiling point, but only if the examining physician is particularly astute, or if the exam includes a psychological evaluation. Normally they go undetected.

However, a good place to detect emotional disturbances is on the job. They are bound to interfere with the individual's work habits, performance, and relations with co-workers. For this reason, companies are advised by experts to make sure that supervisors have at least a rudimentary ability to recognize the kinds of behavior that indicate serious problems.

The classification of mental disorders is, of course, a subject worthy of encyclopedic effort. However, a basic understanding of the two most common problems is sufficient to give you a useful overview.

Anxiety

Anxiety is usually defined as a state of tension associated with apprehension, worry, guilt, insecurity, and a constant need for reassurance. Anxiety should not be confused with ordinary fear or with mild consternation that is in accord with reality. Without some degree of concerned anticipation an individual might be indifferent to significant future events. Fear is considered an appropriate response to real danger. Anxiety, on the other hand, is a reaction that is out of proportion to the actual danger.

Typically, anxiety is accompanied by a host of psychosomatic symptoms such as profuse perspiration, difficulty breathing, gastric disturbances, rapid heartbeat, frequent urination, muscle tension, diarrhea, or high blood pressure. Insomnia is also a reliable indicator, particularly the type that awakens the person during the night. Nightmares may also accompany anxiety.

Depression

A mood characterized by feelings of dejection and gloom, depression usually contains feelings of worthlessness, hopelessness, futility, and guilt. It is more than just melancholia or sadness. "Depression," writes psychiatrist David Viscott, "is a sadness which has lost its relationship to the logical progression of events."

Depression may be mild or severe. In its milder form, it may result directly from a crisis; but people with neurotic tendencies may react inappropriately to emotional experiences. Its more severe manifestation may be innate, determined by biochemical disturbances or genetic predisposition. In its extreme form, depression can occasionally lead to suicide.

According to Dr. Tobias Brocher, director of the Menninger Foundation's Center for Applied Behavioral Science, depression is among the most prevalent and serious of executive problems:

> A high percentage of executives suffer from depression, although it's often hidden. When an executive becomes angry or anxious, often he can't vent his feelings or find legitimate outlets for his aggressions. He may not even admit them to himself. So he becomes depressed as a defense against feelings he doesn't want to recognize in himself.

Both anxiety and depression have been treated with drugs. However, drugs are currently in disfavor because of their dangerous side effects. Depending upon the severity of the situation, various forms of psychiatric intervention are prescribed. This may involve simple counseling, crisis intervention, in-depth psychoanalysis, or one of the newer spin-offs of the human potential movement. Some psychiatrists treat anxiety and depression nutritionally, or with megavitamins, asserting that all mental states have singular biochemical correlates and can therefore be treated physiologically. Then again, mild forms of these difficulties require little more than a good talk with a close friend, a vacation, a change of scene, or a good book. It is important to nip them in the bud, however possible.

—————————— the major stress disorders ——————————

In a very real sense, all functions of mind and body are affected by stress; each encounter depletes some of our adaptation energy, and, when sufficiently powerful, each stressful event will leave some imprint on the nervous system. Some of the consequences are impossible to measure. For example, stress doubtless impairs the functioning of the brain. "Little blood vessels become obstructed and scar," says Dr. Selye, who believes the most obvious losses occur in the brain. "The older you get, the more scar tissue you have. And brain cells don't multiply; so they become more and more blocked."

Experts estimate we use barely a tenth of the brain's potential; many have attributed this to stress. However, we know very little about the brain at the moment, particularly its higher functions. Perhaps future research will reveal that many of our mistakes, confusions, misperceptions, and even social disorder can be traced to the phenomenon of stress.

At the moment, it seems evident that certain diseases endemic to modern society—particularly heart disease—are in some way linked to stress, although there is still much to be learned about the mechanisms responsible. Such disorders are the biggest threats to executives, but they *can* be prevented with alert self-care.

---

self-evaluation: cardiovascular warnings

Ask yourself these questions:

Do you ever feel shortness of breath, as though you can't get enough air in your lungs?
Do you lose breath during physical exertion?
Do you ever have heart palpitations?
Have you ever been told you have high blood pressure?
When your doctor takes your blood pressure, does it fluctuate so much that he has to take it several times?
Has a doctor ever said you have heart trouble?
Have you ever had coronary occlusion, myocardial infarction, or coronary thrombosis?
Do you have chest pains?

> *How severe?*
> *How often?*

Have you ever had an electrocardiogram?

> *When?*
> *What were the results?*

Have you ever had an electrocardiogram while on a treadmill?
Do you get pressure or pain in the chest after exertion?
Has anyone in your family had heart trouble?
Have you ever been told you have an ulcer?
Do you often get severe stomach pains?

Do you seem to need to urinate with excessive frequency?
Does your vision suddenly blur?
Do you have excessive thirst?
Do you get muscle cramps or a stiff neck frequently?
Tension in the shoulders?
Do you often have backaches?
Do you often have headaches?
Have you ever been told you have abnormal blood sugar levels?
Do you have chronic fatigue?
Do you have frequent colds? Viruses? Flus?
Do you have any respiratory problems, such as asthma, sinusitis, allergies, etc?
Do you ever get dizzy spells?
Does your face ever flush?
Do you have trouble sleeping?
Have you suddenly lost weight and strength?

Cardiovascular Disease*

Cardiovascular disease (those afflicting the heart and blood vessels) kills more Americans than all other causes combined. The factors linked to heart disease are so many that no one cause can be identified. "The difficulty surrounding the treatment of coronary heart disease," write cardiologists Meyer Friedman and Ray Rosenman, "is not that we don't know its causes, it is that there are so many causes."

causes of heart disease

Here is a partial list of factors associated with heart disease:

heredity
elevated blood pressure
elevated serum cholesterol
elevated fat levels in blood
diets high in fats and cholesterol
cigarette smoking
obesity
diabetes
personality and behavior (see chapter five)
life changes

*This chapter discusses the causes and symptoms of stress disorders. Treatment is discussed in the next chapter. Prevention in general is the subject of chapters five though nine.

lack of exercise
degree of religious participation
anxiety and neuroticism

Arguments rage as to the degree of impact each factor has. For example, *blood* cholesterol contributes to the formation of obstructions in blood vessels, and it has been assumed that *food* cholesterol—that is, cholesterol taken in through eating—is therefore a cause of atherosclerosis. This, however, has been widely contested. Similarly, exercise has been useful in treating patients with heart problems, but disputes rage over whether or not *lack* of exercise *causes* heart problems. (These controversies will be discussed in chapters seven and six, respectively.)

To some degree, however, the stress reaction is definitely a factor. The fight-or-flight response centers largely around the heart and blood vessels: blood pressure soars, the pulse pounds, the blood is diverted to the limbs and other vital areas, and the blood chemistry changes, fed by the outpouring of adrenal hormones and the intake of fatty substances from the body's stores. In the long run, repeated stimulation of this type can lead to any number of ailments, including heart attack. Certain behavior patterns, which are linked to this syndrome, are described in depth in chapter five. The next two sections discuss the primary areas of cardiovascular disease: atherosclerosis and hypertension.

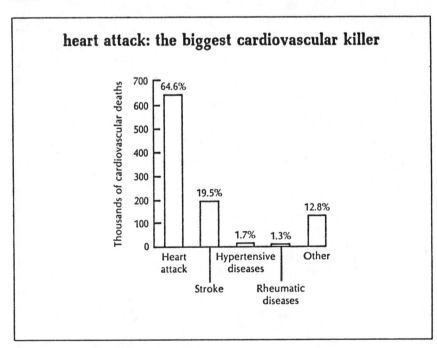

heart attack: the biggest cardiovascular killer

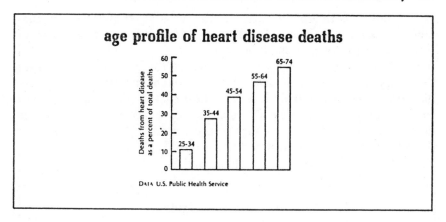

age profile of heart disease deaths

Data U.S. Public Health Service

---
atherosclerosis

Atherosclerosis (sometimes called arteriosclerosis) is an abnormal narrowing of the arteries.

Arteries are structured in three layers. Atherosclerosis begins when the elastic lining between the two innermost layers becomes damaged. Apparently, wounds in the elastic layer are common, occuring even in infancy, for reasons that are not quite clear. Whatever the causes of these little wounds, they leave scars that slightly thicken the artery walls but are quite harmless in themselves. Problems arise when cholesterol and fat irritate the cells in the ruptured area. As more and more particles seep in, the cells multiply. Soon the particles surround the broken area, forming a sort of fatty sheen. Even at this stage, relatively little harm can be done. But if the process continues, the cells will eventually burst, spilling their contents into the surrounding area.

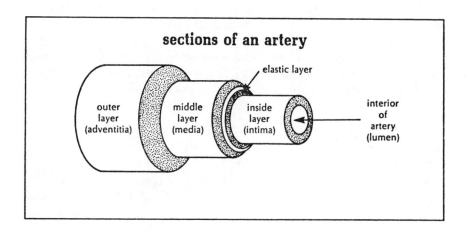

sections of an artery

In defense, the body initiates the process known as *fibrosis,* whereby connective tissue grows in and around the damaged area to seal it off. Ultimately, a plaque is formed that extends into the *lumen,* the hollow part of the artery through which the blood flows, and into the artery wall itself. The plaque gets covered over with a tough, scar-like substance. New blood vessels are formed, extending to the plaque from the outer layers of the artery wall. These new vessels are rather makeshift, so that the plaque rarely receives enough blood. That, plus the interference of excess fat and cholesterol leads to the death of cells in the plaque. The degeneration may lead to bursting.

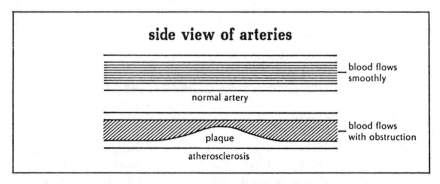

The plaque can be so large that it blocks the blood flowing through the artery. In addition, debris and clotted blood from a ruptured plaque may circulate through the bloodstream; some fragments may be large enough to block a blood vessel. When an artery is blocked, the cells that it serves are starved. Since blockages can occur in any artery, atherosclerosis can lead to damage anywhere in the body.

Stroke

If blockage occurs in arteries feeding the brain, oxygen and nutrients cannot get to the nerve cells. Those cells can die as a result. This is the condition known as a stroke. The part of the body controlled by the damaged nerve cells no longer functions correctly. Paralysis follows. The effects of stroke vary from very slight to severe, and from temporary to permanent.

Angina Pectoris

This occurs when some area of the heart muscle is temporarily deprived of blood. Angina can be mild or unbearably painful. It is usually experienced as a sensation of tightening in the chest or heavy pressure and pain behind the breastbone. Stabbing chest pains and the feeling of suffocation are common. The pain may radiate down either arm (usually the left) or up the neck to the jaws. The pain usually lasts no more than a few minutes, and it most often appears when demands on the heart are excessive—after a very heavy meal, an emotional upset, or vigorous exercise. An affliction worth treating in its own right, angina is a definite precursor of heart attack.

---

those chest pains may not be angina

Dr. Christian Barnard, the renowned surgeon who performed the world's first heart transplant, points out that physicians are frequently confronted by patients who fear that the sharp, stabbing pain on the left side of their chests must be angina.

Dr. Barnard points out that "functional disturbances of the lower end of the esophagus, or gullet, herniation of the stomach through the diaphragm, gallstones, virus infections of the membrane surrounding the heart—these and many other benign conditions commonly give rise to symptoms bearing a very close superficial resemblance to those of ischemic heart pain."

He says that this "cardiac neurosis" is seen most often among depressed and anxious persons. Often, the pain is associated with "a sense of suffocation, light-headedness, and tingling of the fingers and lips," symptoms he associates with the overbreathing brought on by fear and anxiety.

So don't panic if you have a pain in your chest. Your heart may be fine. On the other hand, don't let reassurances such as this convince you that everything is rosy in your chest cavity. Let your doctor make the determination.

Heart Attack

Your heart, like other muscles, needs a supply of blood to stay alive and pumping. The "coronary arteries" branch off from the main artery leaving the heart, to return blood to the heart muscle itself. These coronary arteries can develop atherosclerosis and become clogged. Or, a clot may form elsewhere and lodge in these arteries, blocking blood flow: coronary thrombosis. The muscle cells in the portion of the heart fed by that artery then suffer from *coronary insufficiency,* a shortage of oxygen.

Whether caused by atherosclerotic narrowing of the coronary arteries, or the blockage of those arteries by a clot, the resulting starvation of the heart muscle is a *myocardial infarction,* or heart attack.

Thus, atherosclerosis is the foundation of tragic diseases. When a person dies of a heart attack, we seldom think he or she died of atherosclerosis. But without the arterial plaque growth and subsequent starvation of the heart, it is unlikely that the attack would have occurred.

Detecting Atherosclerosis

Fifty percent or more of American men over twenty-one harbor one or more arterial plaques. In about three percent of American adults, the coronary arteries fail to supply the heart muscles with sufficient nourishment to meet all demands.

Serious atherosclerosis may be present without either the patient or his physician being aware of it. Angina pectoris is one obvious indication, but by that time considerable damage has already been done. Moreover, a person may have a sudden, even fatal heart attack with no prior warning.

Routine physical exams are not sufficient for detecting serious coronary artery disease. Even an electrocardiogram (EKG) often fails to reveal dangerous plaques as long as the heart remains sound. To show up on an EKG, a plaque must block about 90 percent of the artery.

The so-called stress test seems the most reliable at present and is becoming routine in most thorough physicals. EKG and pulse are recorded during a gradually stepped-up workout on a treadmill. Inadequate blood supply to the heart (ischemia) is detectable this way, which enables the doctor to postulate the presence of atherosclerosis.

If the stress test does reveal some abnormality, then an angiogram might be called for. A radio-opaque dye is injected into the coronary arteries; the dye shows up in an X-ray, allowing the physician to observe the actual blood flow through the artery. Angiograms, however, are not used indiscriminately. They require direct entry into the body, and they have been known to precipitate cardiac arrest in high-risk patients. The mortality rate is less than one percent, but doctors use angiograms only when there is a serious problem and a low risk of complications.

Recent advances in cardiac detection include the echo-cardiogram, which uses sound waves; radioactive scanning of the heart; and Holter monitoring, a 24-hour tape recording of heart activity. A new monitor used by persons known to have heart problems can detect abnormalities and give warning of an impending heart attack.

The best examinations combine lab measurements, personal history, and the latest medical statistics in a comprehensive profile. A computer then calculates your statistical likelihood of developing heart problems over the next several years. Using such data, your doctor can make specific recommendations for reducing your risk.

hypertension

Hypertension afflicts one-third of the population over 50. Thirty percent of the cases are undetected. One of the body's responses to stress is to constrict the artery walls. This raises the blood pressure in the artery. When the alarm passes, blood pressure should drop back to normal. But if the stressor is prolonged, even subconsciously, blood pressure can stay abnormally high, decreasing less with each successive alarm, until it stabilizes at a high level—much like a thermostat stuck at a high temperature.

In some cases, hypertension may be attributable to a specific organic cause, such as hardening of the arteries, kidney ailments, excessive secretion of the hormone aldosterone, or kidney obstructions. Each of these conditions can be aggravated by stress. But for 90 percent of hypertensive people there is no apparent cause. This is called "essential hypertension"—either the heart is pumping too much blood, or the blood vessels are too narrow. Again, excessive stress is implicated.

Consequences of Hypertension

Doctors recommend regular monitoring of blood pressure because the disorders associated with it are grave. High blood pressure will make the heart pump harder than normal: it may enlarge, weaken, and lose efficiency. Hypertension can also weaken the arteries, making them less elastic: atherosclerosis may result. Coronary heart disease is three to five times more common among hypertensives.

Weakening of the small blood vessels in the eyes can lead to hemorrhages and blindness. Damage to vessels in the kidneys can destroy the kidney's ability to clear waste from the blood. Risk of stroke is much greater, since the capacity of arteries feeding the brain is reduced.

Detecting Hypertension

In most cases, hypertension itself is painless and produces no visible symptoms. In some cases, dizziness, shortness of breath, flushing of the face, headaches, fatigue, or insomnia might indicate hypertension, but they may just as easily be linked to other problems. Generally speaking, symptoms only appear after hypertension has caused major damage in a vital organ—you can't diagnose it yourself. Because of its virtual invisibility and its tragic consequences, health experts advise regular blood-pressure tests.

The standard (sphygmomanometer) test measures two aspects of blood pressure: systolic and diastolic. Systolic is a measure of the pressure when the heart contracts; diastolic pressure is the heart's dilation phase. It is written systolic/diastolic: 120/80 is considered normal. If readings of 150/90 occur consistently, treatment is usually recommended.

—————————————————————————— **ulcers** —————

Ulcers are inflammatory lesions caused by digestive enzymes eating away at the lining of the stomach or small intestine. Found mainly on the walls of the duodenum and the stomach, they have long been associated with frustration; attacks are known to be triggered by serious losses—deaths, getting fired, divorce, etc. When stress patterns change, the incidence of ulcers also changes.

Interestingly, the notion that ulcers are an essential part of executive life has recently been debunked. Not only do top executives often ride out their careers ulcer-free, but laborers and housewives seem to be cutting in on the lines for antacid tablets.

Back in the Victorian era, 7 of 10 ulcer sufferers were women. By the 1950s, the trend had reversed: 9 of 10 were men. Now, the trend is shifting back: ulcer cases only four times as frequent among men. This may be a consequence of the changing roles of women in the labor market.

Elusive Causes of Ulcers

Cigarette smoking, alcohol, aspirin, and cortisone variations are said to precipitate ulcers, but the relationship is never clearly one of cause and effect. Predisposition to ulcers seems to be inheritable, but no clear pattern has yet been identified.

The discussion invariably comes back to personality and life-style. It is not hard work that is at fault. Rather, it is gnawing unhappiness and dissatisfaction with personal limitations, forcing oneself to strive for things that are really unattainable, or nagging guilt that one is not doing enough.

Psychologists do not all feel that there is any "typical" ulcer personality, but there is general agreement that frustration, tension, anguish, fear, worry, and other disturbing emotions are prime elements. Dr. Robert Collier Page, an international medical consultant to government and industry, recommends analyzing the situations that bring on indigestion or queasiness in the stomach. By noting these stressors you can avoid them, change the way you respond to them, or learn to put them in a more useful perspective.

diabetes

Diabetes is a serious disease, a killer with such grim potential complications as blindness, heart disease, stroke, tuberculosis, kidney failure, and vascular disease. Deficiencies of insulin, the pancreatic hormone responsible for metabolizing glucose, render diabetics unable to absorb enough blood sugar into their cells. The glucose instead accumulates in the blood, depriving the body of its glucose energy source and forcing it to burn stores of fat. That, plus the need for eliminating excess glucose through urination upsets the body's chemistry severely. If the condition is unchecked, the brain will be affected, and diabetic coma will result. Americans have an extraordinary rate of diabetes—25 cases per 1000 persons.

Heredity may play a role; some postulate that diabetics inherit deficiencies of the pancreas. Diet is thought by some to be a causative factor. Stress has also been implicated. It has been shown that stressful situations increase the blood sugar level, and that diabetic patients suffer more severely under stress. If called upon to secrete insulin persistently due to chronically high sugar levels, the pancreas may weaken, resulting in permanent insulin deficiency.

Detecting Diabetes

The trick is to catch diabetes in time. Ninety percent of its victims are afflicted between the ages of 35 and 60. The form of the disease that begins in youth is fast-developing and requires regular insulin shots to control. The adult variation is usually easier to deal with, but is insidiously slow to develop and difficult to spot.

---

diabetes warnings

Be on the alert for these factors:

*hereditary inclination—if your parents or grandparents were diabetic,
   you are a likely candidate*
unexplained loss of strength and weight
excessive thirst
frequent urination
sudden change in, or blurring of, vision
20 percent or more overweight

If you have any of these symptoms or tendencies, see your doctor. Even in the absence of warning signs, a routine urine or blood test should be part of every physical exam. If your doctor suspects that you might have diabetes, he will order a "glucose tolerance test." This test must be done after you have fasted for at least eight hours. Then, after drinking some glucose, your blood is tested every half hour for four to six hours. In this way, your response to sugar can be monitored for abnormalities.

headaches

Action-oriented, competitive, aggressive people tend to develop muscular tension. Their muscles are, in a sense, never at rest; they are in a semicontracted state even when the individual is not working.

Among sedentary workers, the tension usually resides in the back and shoulders, which is why so many executives get such delight from a good rubdown. Sometimes the tension will affect the muscles of the scalp and neck, leading to tension headache. Unfortunately, this sort of tension is self-perpetuating. The pain makes you tense the muscles still further, which leads to more pain, and so on.

Dr. Robert Collier Page offers the following personality profile of headache-prone executives:

> You are, by nature, something of a perfectionist. You worry a little more than others about the good opinion of society—or of your own conscience. You do not laugh things off easily. If you are "out of sorts" one day and unable to do what you consider to be your duty, you are unable to say, "Ah well, I'll make up for it tomorrow!" ... Most of us learn to forgive ourselves, but you cannot. Most of us find it necessary to "unwind" occasionally—forget the demands of perfection—and "waste time" just relaxing and having fun. You cannot do this either, with grace. Even on vacation you are worrying about your performance in the eyes of society (or your conscience). You can't let go. Any attempt on your part to thumb your nose at your conscience—to be yourself without being self-conscious about it—brings terrible retribution: a headache.

Before treating a regularly recurring headache, first determine whether it is a migraine (see next section) or a simple tension headache. The treatment will differ radically; a cocktail, for example, might be a good strategy for a tension headache, but it could aggravate a vascular headache. Some doctors advise keeping a headache diary. Note the date and time of onset and remission, what you were doing when the headache started, what happened the day before, what you ate, and the nature of the pain. The notes may be important in diagnosing the cause of your headaches. Physicians say that patients often have sound intuitive feelings about what triggered an attack.

─────────────────── **migraine headaches** ───────────────────

Not to be confused with ordinary tension headaches, migraines strike with such fury that one sufferer, Thomas Jefferson, was moved to write: "The art of life is the avoiding of pain." Throbbing head, teary eyes, blurry vision, and waves of nausea make the slightest attack unbearable.

The pain is caused by the dilation of blood vessels in the scalp, thus technically qualifying migraines as a cardiovascular ailment. Local inflammation may accompany the swollen vessels, and certain biochemical changes are also postulated. About half an hour before the pain sets in, most migraine sufferers experience a so-called aura—blind spots, numbness in the limbs or lips, sensitivity to light or noise, and often hallucinations.

Usually the pain comes on one side of the head (*migraine* stems from the Greek for "half skull"), occurring in many cases at the same time on the same day each week. The pain can last 15 minutes or several days; it may come as often as twice a week. Women are three times as likely to have migraines as men, but *cluster* headaches, so called because they strike repeatedly over the course of several hours, most often affect men

Causes

Several factors are said to trigger attacks of migraines: heavy lifting, estrogen hormones in birth-control pills, carbon monoxide, alcohol, and certain food substances, such as chocolate, ripened cheese, citrus fruits, vinegar, nuts, and monosodium glutamate. Stress, of course, is a major causal or aggravating factor.

Dr. Harold G. Wolff, one of the pioneer researchers in the field of psychosomatic medicine, determined that migraine sufferers are typically insecure. Their feelings of worthlessness make them drive hard and overburden themselves with thankless responsibilities, which they pursue compulsively. Interestingly, it is not during stressful times that migraines tend to come. "Instead," reports author Walter McQuade, "it is when the pressure lifts and they are, so to speak, off duty. Sunday is a notorious migraine day."

The symptoms of migraine can be both insidious and alarming. In some instances they may mimic more serious disorders. If you are in doubt as to whether you are a migraine sufferer, it is strongly recommended that you discuss your symptoms with a doctor. A headache diary can be very useful to him for your diagnosis.

disorders of the immune system

The human body is equipped with a defense system so complex and elegant that the machinations of the Pentagon seem like a touch-football game by comparison. The immune system, which uses many weapons (such as antibodies), is well equipped to distinguish between self and non-self. Any foreign invader is quickly recognized and dealt with through a remarkable attack-and-devour strategy. When the immune system is faulty, or if it fails to act quickly enough, a wide variety of diseases can occur.

Infections, viruses, flus, and colds, of course, are common consequences, and the fact that run-down people are especially susceptible to these breakdowns has led scientists to postulate that stress may be an important factor. Asks Hans Selye, rhetorically, "If a microbe is in or around us all the time and yet causes no disease until we are exposed to stress, what is the 'cause' of our illness, the microbe or the stress?"

Emotional problems stimulate the hypothalamus, which alerts the pituitary to signal the release of adrenal hormones called *glucocorticoid.* With an excess of these hormones the body apparently produces fewer antibodies, and the inflammatory response is inhibited.

One of the maladies most clearly associated with stress and with an out-of-whack immune system is allergy. Allergens are, of course, legion, and many of us are sensitive to some but not others. What happens, essentially, is that the body is being antagonized by its own protective mechanisms. It responds to the allergen by mobilizing certain chemicals (notably histamine) which cause tissues to swell, mucus secretions to rise, and airway passages in the lungs to contract. Hence, the typical asthmatic or allergic response—sneezing, wheezing, itching, etc. Attacks are worse under stress, and often don't occur at all in its absence. Some experiments have even shown that allergy sufferers respond with classic symptoms at the mere sight, or thought, of the allergen, even when it is not physically present.

Rheumatoid arthritis and ulcerative colitis are both thought to be caused by immune system deficiencies, although the connection is not yet clear. Scientists suspect that the inflammation and lesions characteristic of each illness may be caused by "autoimmunity"; failure to distinguish self from non-self leads to the manufacture of antibodies that work against the body's own tissues. Both maladies flare up under stress.

Cancer

While the cause of cancer is still a matter of intense scientific inquiry, stressful life events and general patterns of disappointment, loneliness, and unhappiness have been found to correlate with the incidence of cancer. The immune system has recently been accused of being a possible mediating factor.

According to this theory, cellular mutations are a regular occurrence, but a healthy immune system destroys the mutants before they can multiply. Some mutant cells survive, multiply, and become tumors. Here an enemy is mistaken for a friend and allowed to live inside the body.

Breakthroughs are constantly being made in the battle against cancer. In the meantime, doctors agree, many deaths can be prevented by regular examinations. Cancer of the colon, for example, can be detected by sigmoidoscopic examinations of the lower intestine. Regular examinations can detect prostate cancer in men, and a regular "PAP" smear of the cervix can detect cervical cancer in women. Women should also pay careful attention to changes in menstruation and have a regular pelvic examination in order to minimize the risk of cancer of the uterus or ovaries.

Breast cancer afflicts some 90,000 victims each year and is a leading cause of death among women 40 to 44 years of age. It is curable if detected early. Doctors advise that all women examine their breasts thoroughly once a month, preferably just after the menstrual period, to look for lumps, thickenings, or nodules. While irregularities are a normal occurrence, the monthly self-examination will teach you what is normal for you, thus enabling you to detect variations if they should arise. Most changes are *not* signs of cancer, but they should be reported to a doctor immediately so that a professional diagnosis can be made.

---

self-examination of breasts

Your doctor will be able to show you how to examine your breasts. For an illustrated pamphlet describing self-examination procedures, write to Life Extension Institute, 1185 Avenue of the Americas, New York, N.Y. 10036.

In addition to self-examinations, regular check-ups by a physician are recommended. If you are over 50, if you have had cancer or lumps on the breast or a family history of breast cancer, or if you are over 30 and have been unable to become pregnant, then a *mammography* is called for. This is a special X-ray designed to pinpoint abnormal tissue growths before they can be detected manually. It is the best diagnostic device available.

—— **recommended reading: chapters 1-3** ——

Body and Antibody: A Report on the New Immunology, David Wilson (New York: Knopf, 1971).

Emotional Health and the World of Work, Harry Levinson (New York: Harper & Row, 1964).

Future Shock, Alvin Toffler (New York: Random House, 1970).

Heart Attack: You Don't Have to Die, Christian Barnard (New York: Delacorte, 1972).

Man Alone, Josephson and Josephson, eds. (New York: Dell, 1973).

Mind as Healer, Mind as Slayer, Kenneth R. Pelletier (New York: Delacorte, 1977).

Occupational Stress, Hahn et al. (Springfield, Ill: Charles C. Thomas, 1974).

"Recent Evidence Supporting Psychologic and Social Risk Factors for Coronary Disease," David Jenkins, *New England Journal of Medicine,* April 29 and May 6, 1976 (vol. 294, nos. 18 and 19).

Stress, Walter McQuade and Ann Aikman (New York: Dutton, 1974).

"Stress," Kathy Slobogin, *New York Times Magazine,* November 20, 1977. "What Stress Can Do To You," Walter McQuade, *Fortune,* January 1972.

Stress and Disease, Harold G. Wolff (Springfield, Ill: Charles C. Thomas, 1968).

Stress without Distress, Hans Selye (Philadelphia: Lippincott, 1974).

The Stress of Life, Hans Selye (New York: McGraw-Hill, 1956).

The Visible Hand, Alfred Chandler (Cambridge, Mass.: Harvard U. P., 1977).

Urban Stress, Glass and Singer (New York: Academic Press, 1972).

You Can Fight Cancer and Win, Jane E. Brody (New York: Quadrangle, 1977).

Your Heart, Likoff and Segal (Philadelphia: Lippincott, 1972).

executive health strategies

medical care: the first line of defense

---

self-evaluation: health checkpoints

1. Have you had a complete physical examination within the last year?
2. Were you given specific instructions by your physician? Do you follow them to the letter?
3. Have you had any serious ailments in the last five years?
4. How many days of work have you missed because of illness this year?
5. Do you ever use aspirin or other headache remedies? Approximately how often?
6. Do you ever use tranquilizers or sleeping pills? How often?
7. Other medication, prescribed or nonprescribed?
8. Do you smoke cigarettes? How many per day?
9. How much do you drink?
10. Do you see your doctor when symptoms appear or do you ignore them hoping they will go away?
11. Do you think of your health at times when you have no discernible illness?

—————————————————— **the annual physical** ——————

The trend toward preventive medicine has made annual physical examinations almost standard policy in most large corporations, even though their cost-effectiveness has sometimes been challenged.

Proponents of exams point out that the big killers—heart problems and other degenerative diseases—are "silent sicknesses," because they display few discernible signs until they have progressed past the danger point. Modern advances in diagnostic instruments have made it possible to detect these disorders early enough to treat them effectively. I.B.M. claims that one-third of its employee exams turned up medical problems that the subject had been unaware of.

Others feel that exams do not yield enough disease detection to be worth the cost. In most diseases, the argument goes, treatment is not practical before symptoms have developed to the point where the victim recognizes them. In addition, most patients (and many doctors) pay little attention to symptoms until discomfort appears.

Harvard endocrinologist Dr. Richard Spark is one of a number of eminent physicians who oppose regular exams. "The annual physical examination has proved to be little more than an elaborate and expensive ritual," he contends.

Dr. Spark points to a seven-year study at Kaiser-Permanente's prepaid health plan, wherein 5000 people were urged to have annual physicals while another group was not. The first group—which had been examined about three times as often—showed no appreciable difference in health. Its death rate *was* slightly lower, but more of its members had chronic diseases.

Dr. Morris Collen, the physician responsible for this study, disagrees with Dr. Spark's conclusion. He feels that the main purpose of an exam is to detect "potentially postponable" illnesses such as heart disease. According to Dr. Collen, the results of the Kaiser experiment show that "if one has a checkup every year or two at age 35 and thereafter, directed at postponable diseases, the mortality rate *from those diseases* after seven years is approximately 50 percent of what it would have been without exams."

Spark counters by claiming that physicals instill "the reassuring feeling that since all systems have been checked, the individual will remain healthy for at least one more year or 12,000 miles, whichever comes first." But the threat of patient complacency is perhaps trivial compared with the value of early detection and genuine education. Prevention-oriented physicians also cite the advantages of establishing a personal relationship with a physician, with whom the individual can subsequently consult if symptoms do appear.

The benefits of regular exams are not only physical; many companies now make psychological evaluations part of the process. Dr. Robert R. J. Hilker, president of the Occupational Medical Association feels that "the greatest amount of job dysfunction is caused not by physical illness but behavioral problems." He adds that the average family doctor seldom takes the time to probe and doesn't understand corporate life, a good argument for using a doctor who specializes in executives. Even in the absence of formal interviews, the physical exams have definite psychological advantages: "You go back to your routine in a surer state of mind," says Dr. Richard Winter, director of Executive Health Examiners.

corporate physicals

Fortune magazine surveyed 130 of the largest companies in the United States and found that 66 of the 72 respondents provided regular physicals for their employees. Most of the companies provided the exams only for managers and professionals, while about one-fourth cover all employees. Of those with an opinion on the question, more than three times as many felt that the physicals resulted in less absenteeism. The overwhelming majority of employees, the survey found, will eagerly accept the company's offer of free examinations.

A growing number of companies—68 percent of those offering exams—conduct them on their own premises, at costs ranging from under $100 to over $300 per person. (Outside exams can be more expensive.)

in-house medical units

According to Executive Health Examiners, in-house medical units have these important advantages:

prompt handling of emergencies
reduced absenteeism (an employee who is slightly under the weather may not stay home if he knew he could see a competent expert on the job)
reduced Workman's Compensation costs
reduced necessity of sending employees to hospitals for lab tests
experts to counsel about chronic risk factors such as stress, overweight, alcohol, etc.
reduced time lost due to employees leaving early

ten of the top clinics for annual checkups

Clinic	Address/Telephone	Cost	Time Required	Recommended Advance Reservation	Special Services
Vincent Astor Diagnostic Service	New York Hospital Cornell Medical Center 525 E. 68th St. New York, N.Y. (212) 879-9000	$90 basic fee	3 hours	4-6 weeks	Attention to signs of stress, pulmonary tests for smokers
Benjamin Franklin Clinic	330 S. 9th St. Philadelphia, Pa. (215) 829-3402	$235 (corporate rate; $160 for some younger employees), $300 (individual referrals)	3-4 hours	4 weeks	
Cleveland Clinic	220 E. 93rd St. Cleveland, Ohio (216) 229-2200	$120-$180	One full day (or two half-days)	6-8 weeks	
The Executive Health Examiners	777 Third Ave. New York, N.Y. (212) 486-8900	$150 average	3 hours	2-4 weeks	Pulmonary analysis Coronary risk profile cross-country affiliates
Lahey Clinic	605 Commonwealth Ave. Boston, Mass. (617) 261-2200	$270 for initial series, $160 per annual follow-up	3-day battery of exams, 1-day checkups annually thereafter	4-6 weeks	Stress EKG, psychiatric consultation when indicated

Continued on following page.

Clinic	Address/Telephone	Cost	Time Required	Recommended Advance Reservation	Special Services
Mayo Clinic	200 S.W. 1 St. Rochester, Minn. (507) 282-2511	$200-$400	One full day	One year	
Ochsner Clinic	1514 Jefferson Hwy. Jefferson Parish New Orleans, La. (504) 834-7070	$75-$300	One full day	2-6 weeks	Pulmonary tests for smokers
Palo Alto Medical Clinic	300 Homer Ave. Palo Alto, Calif. (415) 321-4121	$200 for full exam	One day, unless further tests indicated	2-4 weeks	
Scott-White Clinic	Scott-White Hospital Temple, Tex. (817) 778-4451	$235.50 average for over-40 patients	Two days, on average	2 weeks, earlier in summer	Special attention to recent overseas returnees
Scripps Clinic & Research Foundation	476 Prospect La Jolla, Calif. (714) 459-2390	$215-$280	2-3 days	Sufficient time to return pre-admission questionnaire	
Life Extension Institute	1185 Ave. of Americas New York, N.Y. (212) 575-8300	$100-$300	2-3½ hours	2-4 weeks	Cross-country affiliates Risk factors profile

return-to-work checkups
preplacement screening examinations
*personal relationship with an available expert where the employee
spends his day*

Another advantage, aside from long-range costs, is that clinics
catering to businessmen have been swamped in recent years, cutting
severly into the time of physicians and creating waiting lists as long
as eight weeks. At deluxe facilities like the Mayo Clinic, executive
physicans must be booked a year in advance.

The Importance of Regular Examinations

Most advocates of physicals do not insist that everyone be examined
annually. According to Fortune writer Walter McQuade, the consensus
on frequency of exams is about as follows:

20s and early 30s (if healthy) ....*every 5 years*
35–45 ....*every 2–3 years*
over 45 .... *every year*

The older one gets, of course, the more time stress has had to undermine the system. "A motor car doesn't suddenly cease running because
of old age," writes Dr. Selye. "It stops because of the failure of some part
that has worn out. It is the same with people. Under continuous stress
—either mental or physical—some vital body part gives way, leading
to a variety of illnesses, and eventually to death."

It is particularly important for executives over 40 to be examined
every year, because the signs of serious illness are more discernible
then. Says Dr. Russell Roth, president of the American Medical Association, "At 40, the yield of useful information you can act on starts to go
way up." Middle-aged businessmen, especially the sedentary type,
could be living dangerously if they pass up an annual exam.

New Early-Warning Systems

The businessman who skips next year's physical is likely to lose out on
advances most experts expect will be common soon. The treadmill
electrocardiogram, for example, may not have been available at the
time of your last physical. Dr. John McCann, chairman of Life Extension Institute, predicts that his executive clients will be wearing portable electrocardiograms at their desks before long, a major improvement
over current technology.

Computers have also found their way into the examination room. In some clinics, personal medical history (incorporating as many as two-hundred questions) plus all relevant findings from the doctor's exam are fed into a computer. A personal health forecast is calculated, including present and future risks for every major cause of death, and revealing among other things your statistical likelihood of dying in the next few years.

---

automated prognosis

Here is a summary of a three-page computer printout for a fictitious patient, prepared by Interhealth, Inc., a San Diego affiliate of Life Extension Institute.

Mary Jones, age 50, is told by the computer that her chances of dying in the next ten years are 43 percent greater than her statistical counterpart. The average woman of 50 has a 6.6 percent chance of dying in the next decade (6650 deaths out of 100,000 people)—Mary's is 9.5 percent. The computer reports that her current "risk age" is 55. In effect, she is "clinically" five years older than her chronological age.

Mary has twice the average risk of heart disease, five times the average risk of a fatal auto accident, and double the chance of getting cirrhosis of the liver.

The Health Risk Profile tells Mary to be particularly aware of certain risk factors: If she can reduce her blood pressure to 120/80 or less this will probably add .3 years to her life. If she can stop smoking (or cut down significantly), this could add 2.4 years. If she can reduce or eliminate alcohol consumption, another 2.2 years could be added. Cholesterol, exercise, weight, and other factors are also listed, offering Mary Jones a total of 8.0 years that might be added to her expected life span if she follows specific recommendations. According to the optimistic computer, Mary could reduce her chances of dying in the next ten years by half—to a mere 5 percent, which is better than average for a woman her age.

The Personal Touch—Your Own Doctor

Although such innovations are worth keeping up with, physicians are careful to point out the importance of traditional examining procedures. "Nothing of that sort can replace a personalized examination," says Dr. Alexander Rush, medical director of the Benjamin Franklin Clinic in Philadelphia.

It is easy to underrate the doctor's manual and visual examination, in which he checks everything from eyes to reflexes. Specialists say this routine is more important than any single mechanical test, and should take less than an hour, including time for a rectal sigmoidoscopic exam (to detect signs of colonic cancer).

The personal touch is one of the advantages of in-house medical programs, which are fast taking the place of the almost extinct family physician. In the absence of a family or corporate physician, the executive is strongly advised to find a physician or clinic that he trusts, and return there for each physical. By so doing, you are enabling the doctor to notice subtle changes that develop between visits—changes in your demeanor or your complexion, for example, that might be undetectable by a machine or someone unfamiliar with you.

---

the basic physical examination

Complete physical exams for executives generally have five to eight alternatives to choose from. These vary in number of variables investigated and time spent with the patient. Costs range from $100 to $400 depending on the quality of service desired and the amount of attention required. The following services are usually provided:

Review of personal and family health history This is increasingly being done by computer in advance of the actual physical. In this way the examining physician can study a complete analysis of hereditary and personal variables before the subject even arrives.

Complete manual physical examination Stethoscope, reflex tests, blood pressure, manual probing, and all the familiar procedures right down to the tongue depressor should be provided.

Spirometer Especially important for smokers, this tests "vital capacity" and can reveal a proclivity to emphysema and other respiratory obstructions.

Eye tests To examine near and distant vision, lateral and vertical vision, and color vision.

Test for glaucoma New machines measure interocular pressure with nothing but a puff of air to touch the eye.

Hearing test with an audiometer

Chest X-rays To detect abnormalities in heart and lungs.

Proctosigmoidoscopic exam To detect signs of intestinal disorders, cancer of the colon, ulcerative colitis, and other rectal and bowel illnesses.

Upper gastrointestinal survey (GI series) An X-ray exam of the esophagus, stomach, and small intestine.

Stool examination

Thyroid function test

PAP test and mammography for women

Blood tests To analyze serum cholesterol, blood sugar, urea nitrogen, uric acid, calcium, protein, phosphate, hemoglobin, red and white cells, and other elements.

Urinalysis For sugar, albumin, occult blood, pH, and other factors.

Twelve-lead electrocardiogram (EKG) To analyze the electric currents that traverse the heart while the patient is at rest.

Triglyceride determination   This test reveals important aspects of fat metabolism associated with heart disease.

Lipid profile   A three-part test for blood fats.

Exercise tolerance stress test   Constant monitoring of EKG (and usually blood pressure and pulse rate) during a programmed workout on a treadmill.

Test results will usually be compiled within two weeks and sent to you with a written explanation, signed by your examining physician. Ideally, you should then meet with the physician. A computer analysis of quantifiable portions of your exam may also be made available. To assure confidentiality, your signed permission should be required before any data can be shown to any person or organization. Most clinics providing executives' annual exams do not provide treatment; referrals are made, along with a complete evaluation.

——— two medical services companies: a profile ———

The demand for professional examiners' service has skyrocketed in recent years, as have the complexity and depth of medical technology. Corporate medical service companies have evolved to offer the most efficient and accurate examination techniques in a context expressly designed to meet the needs of business people. Perhaps more than any other new health practice, these comprehensive service outfits reflect the holistic approach to total health that has become so central to modern medicine.

In the next few pages, we will survey two giants in the field of company medical services: Life Extension Institute and Executive Health Examiners. While there are now many such services, these two have been selected as being both representative and exemplary of the best available.

Life Extension Institute
HQ: 1185 Avenue of the Americas
New York, N.Y. 10036
(212) 575-8300

The biggest and oldest of its kind, LEI has been in business since 1913 and is now a Dunn & Bradstreet corporation. Every year its 900 associated physicians perform 40,000 exams, 80 percent of which are paid for by corporations. LEI has three facilities in New York, several in

California (under the name Preventive Medicine Medical Group, Inc.), and others in Denver, Chicago, Philadelphia, and Baltimore.

The LEI staff is drawn largely from the fields of occupational medicine, preventive medicine, and public health. Its specialists cover virtually all areas, and are backed up by nurses, paramedical personnel, and technicians. All examinee records are kept in confidential, active files for three years, after which they are stored on microfilm. Female examining physicians are available on request.

---

life extension institute services

In addition to basic examinations, LEI provides the following services:

Innoculation and Immunization International Certificates of Vaccination for influenza, smallpox, typhoid, tetanus, cholera, plague, yellow fever, or polio.

Dental Services Emergency care, preventive and diagnostic exams, treatment.

Occupational Medicine On-site safety and health surveys to help companies maintain safe work environments and comply with the Occupational Safety and Health Act.

Medical Consultative Services To advise retirement committees and disability boards, review health-care plans, and provide claim-control assistance.

StayWell Health Risk Profile Computerized report described above.

Medical Departments and Emergency Care Staffs and manages medical departments on the premises of client companies. "Multiple subscriber" departments are available for companies wishing to share a facility with another company.

Health Education Program An attempt to "bridge the gap between health information and health practices": programs to educate clients in forming healthful habits.

Individual programs include:

Employees Assistance Program To retain valued employees who become afflicted with medical or emotional/behavioral problems.

Health Counseling Consultations with a health educator for particular problems, especially in areas such as smoking, alcoholism, weight control, etc.

Basic Life Support Training Programs Training in cardiopulmonary resuscitation for use in emergencies.

Organized Programs Individually designed group programs for education on subjects such as hypertension, cardiovascular risks, nutrition, drugs, office safety, cancer, aging and retirement, and stress (to be discussed separately in the next chapter).

The Executive Health Examiners Group
HQ: 777 Third Avenue
New York, N.Y. 10017
(212) 486-8900

Founded in 1959 and privately owned, EHE has over 850 corporate clients ranging from Allied Chemical to Xerox. Their professional staff are all board certified; no paramedics are used. Like LEI, EHE has excellent facilities and the most up-to-date equipment and testing procedures. It is staffed by an interdisciplinary team of specialists committed to preventive medicine. The full-time physicians at their New York headquarters are all internists.

EHE offers essentially the same examination services as LEI, and at comparable prices. EHE maintains medical staffs in New York; Stamford, Connecticut; and Morristown, New Jersey. A network of affiliated medical specialists in more than 500 cities provides EHE with close to 600 associate examiners. The associated examiners provide the same services for the examinee as are offered in the New York facility, but at a slightly higher rate. They use the same forms, which are all processed in New York to insure quality control and accurate record keeping.

A corporation may send one person or its entire employee population for examinations; EHE offers lower fees to organizations sending 20 or more employees.

---

executive health examiners services

Through member organizations, EHE provides a host of services in addition to its physical examinations.

EHE/Executive Health Examiners Conducts periodic and preplacement examinations throughout the U.S. and abroad. Large clients often have a medical director who uses EHE services as an adjunct to his or her own. If there is no medical director, EHE works with management to develop specific programs. As contract operator of clinics and medical departments of the client's premises, it provides the personnel, equipment, medications, insurance, and all other essentials. EHE purchases medication at bulk rate, and provides malpractice and liability insurance, lab tests at no additional cost, medical staff supervision, periodic inspections, and education and consultation services.

EHE/Healthscan Corp. When comprehensive examinations are impractical, EHE offers low-cost exams for groups on the client's premises. Conducted by paramedical staff, exams include a medical history questionnaire and a series of basic screening tests. The patient receives a computer-generated report of test results and recommendations.

EHE/Occumed Programs, Inc. Consultations, mass examinations, and long-term medical surveillance are offered to help companies comply with the Federal Occupational Safety and Health Act, designed according to each company's needs.

EHE/StressControl Systems, Inc. One of the pioneers in corporate stress-management programs, this service offers a broad range of methods, described in chapter five.

In addition, EHE provides education and life-style programs. Usually conducted in companies where EHE has on-site health units, these include cardiopulmonary resuscitation, first aid training, physical fitness programs, and seminars on such topics as diabetes, heart disease, smoking, stress, etc.

——— **medical exams and job placement** ———

In many companies physical examinations are a part of standard employment procedures. Generally speaking, this serves two purposes: to see if a new person's health has any bearing on his or her ability to do the job, and to establish a baseline set of health records for the new employee, a first step in any ongoing medical program.

The use of medical data in placement decisions has stirred controversy. Many employees refuse to take company-sponsored physicals for fear that the results may prejudice their advancement. More than a third of one Fortune survey's respondants admitted turning down candidates for key executive positions because of their health. To assuage those fears, employees are generally told that their medical records will not be made available to the personnel department.

The dilemma centers on whether the doctor's responsibility is to the patient or the employer. Medical ethics dictate that the doctor should serve the patient in confidence unless his health poses a legitimate danger to the community. But this is seldom a clear-cut situation within a corporation.

Dr. Leon Warshaw, medical director of the Equitable Life Assurance Society, quoted in *Fortune,* asks:

> Could I let a man be promoted into a job knowing that he's likely to collapse in it? My obligation to the company tells me I can't. But if I block one promotion for the good of the company, even if it is for the good of the patient's own health as well, inevitably it would become known, and the total program would go down the drain because no one would trust me after that. A periodic health check has to be intended for the benefit of the individual.

In at least 20 states, new laws have been passed prohibiting discrimination in employment because of disability. All of these affect preplacement exams, the hiring of new employees, and promotion policies. Any corporation, especially if it has facilities in more than one state, should have its legal service check out the appropriate laws; they vary from one state to the next. According to Executive Health Examiners, the following general guidelines should be followed:

It is now illegal to discriminate for health reasons except where the condition interferes with the individual's ability to do the job. This applies to hiring, promotions, transfers, discharges, and retirements.

Certain common problems are not protected under the laws: alcohol and drug abuse, communicable diseases, and external conditions not caused by underlying disease.

how to choose a doctor

Choosing a doctor (or a hospital) could be a decision second only in importance to your choice of a spouse.

"One of the best ways to choose doctors is first to choose a good hospital and then choose the appropriate doctor on its staff," writes Dr. G. Timothy Johnson in his new book, *Doctor! What You Should Know About Health Care Before You Call a Physician* (McGraw-Hill). Call the secretary to the department chairman at a reputable hospital and ask for the names of staff members. Ask for recommendations from friends, neighbors, and business associates; if you are moving, your present family doctor, or your company doctor, may have some leads.

If you have several hospitals to choose from, be sure the one you select is accredited by the Joint Commission on Accreditation of Hospitals—this indicates that minimal standards of care are being met. (Check with the hospital administration or write the JCAH: 837 North Michigan Avenue, Chicago, Ill. 60611.) So-called teaching hospitals usually have up-to-date physicians and the best equipment and facilities. Otherwise, look to nonprofit community hospitals, which are generally preferable to privately owned or government-operated institutions.

Regardless of hospital affiliations, check the doctor's credentials. To a great extent your final choice will be based on how you get along with the physician as a person; but don't let compatibility outweigh qualifications.

doctor hunting

Here are additional points for choosing a doctor:
You can be reasonably sure a specialist has had adequate training if he is board certified in his field.

Membership in an honorary college is another indication of achievement. (FACS, for example, means "Fellow in the American College of Surgeons.")

A doctor who teaches at a university is also usually a good bet; the number of years spent in residency is often very important.

The Health Research Group has recently published *A Consumer's Directory of Prince Georges County (Md.) Doctors,* the first of its kind. The publication lists doctors' names, fees, office hours, amount of time scheduled for each patient, education, board certification, teaching and hospital affiliation, whether drugs are prescribed by their generic names, whether patients are advised of possible side effects; whether birth control is prescribed, and how the doctor feels about abortion. More than a dozen such directories have sprung up around the country.

Don't underestimate your personal reactions. Have a talk with the doctor; see if you relate well to one another on a personal basis. Beware of impressive technology with an assembly-line manner.

Be leery of excessive enthusiasm about new medications. Doctors may look for quick, easy cures and use drugs without paying proper attention to side effects.

Be alert for doctors who have itchy scalpel fingers. It is widely acknowledged that too many doctors shove patients into surgery unnecessarily, or prematurely. If you are not totally convinced surgery is necessary, insist on further testing or seek consultation with another doctor. On the other hand, avoid the cynical attitude that all doctors are charlatans. The best approach is not "shopping around," but to establish a reliable personal relationship.

Virtually every physician is properly trained. But sincerity, wisdom, and the ability to give unselfishly are unteachable. These are the qualities to look for in your doctor.

The best doctor is also something of an educator. Some can detect pathological symptoms but cannot teach patients to cultivate good health. Does your doctor take the time to talk to you about your work, family life, exercise, and diet? Will he explain his recommendations? Is he patient with his patients, or is he always in a hurry?

Above all, remember that no doctor owns a magic wand. His ability to keep *you* healthy is mainly determined by *your own* attitudes, habits, and willingness to cooperate.

self-care

You can take care of yourself better than your doctor can, say self-care advocates. Self-care is the latest wave in a tide of health "consumerism" that began in the late 1960s. Taking your health in your own hands may not be as chancy as it sounds. Many physicians are now sold on self-care, even though it could eventually reduce their daily case loads.

Knowing when you should see a doctor, though, is an important part of the whole self-care movement.

Self-care fans maintain that day-to-day life-style is a better yardstick of physical condition than even the most complete battery of tests. "Habit control" is the first step they recommend for a happier, longer, and less doctored life.

A lengthy study of 7000 adults in California recently gave habit control a huge boost. Those practicing at least six or seven good health habits from age 45 on lived an average of 11 years longer than those only practicing two or three. The habits: no smoking, moderate drinking, seven or eight hours of sleep a night, regular meals, daily breakfast, keeping normal weight, and exercising.

But habit control is just the beginning of self-care. With stethoscopes, otoscopes (for ear exams), blood-pressure cuffs, and other medical gear, you can measure your own pulse, respiration, and blood pressure, pap smears, learn cardiopulmonary resuscitation and the Heimlich maneuver (for blocked throats), and treat food poisoning.

For information on self-care, write to National Self-Help Clearinghouse, 184 Fifth Avenue, New York, N.Y. 10010; Center for Medical Consumers & Health Care Information, 410 E. 62nd Street, New York, N.Y. 10021; and Health Activation Network, P. O. Box 7268, Arlington, Va. 22207.

---

smoking and health

Medical care is the first line of defense, but the *best* defense is a good offense. While doctors may argue about the possible dangers of cholesterol, vitamin deficiencies, and lack of exercise, when it comes to tobacco addiction, there is little disagreement. Cutting down may be one of your most valuable steps in preventive medicine.

The familiar Surgeon General's warning on cigarette packages is a mild slap on the wrist compared to the admonitions of other medical authorities. Research shows that lung cancer, which accounts for 20 percent of all cancers and kills nine of every ten victims, is almost completely avoidable by the individual who gives up smoking. Moderate smokers have eight times the amount of lung cancer as nonsmokers, and heavy smokers have 20 times the risk. It is a rare abstainer who gets the disease.

Smoking increases the risk of pneumonia and also emphysema, a serious lung disorder for which there is no known cure. In this malady the lung cells are so stretched that their elasticity is lost and they cannot properly expel air. Compounding the problem, cigarette smoking also interferes with the body's ability to carry oxygen.

Heavy smoking increases the risk of heart attack three to ten times. Nicotine apparently causes a sharp release of adrenalin; heartbeat increases, and blood pressure rises. Smoking also is thought to help precipitate the convulsion of muscle contractions known as ventricular fibrillation, resulting in cardiac arrest.

The danger of heart attack is further increased in smokers because nicotine stimulates the sympathetic nervous system to overproduce epinephrine and norepinephrine, which hastens the blood-clotting process and damages the arterial walls. In addition, says Dr. George Leonard, senior pathologist at a New Orleans hospital, "the continual jolt from nicotine drives the heart to perhaps 20 extra beats per minute in the heavy smoker. This may amount to ten million extra beats every year (adding an extra year on 'living' in every 3 1/2)."

Studies have shown that people who smoke a pack or more a day are 10 to 15 times as likely to have coronary artery thickening. They also have a 20 percent greater incidence of stroke.

Kicking the Habit

Essentially, there are two ways to quit smoking: cold turkey or tapering off.

Of the former, Dr. Robert Collier Page says:

> If you approach it as a crucial battle that you *must* come out of as the victor, you will see how quickly you begin to lose that urge to light up. Remember that you are trying to kick a type of addiction—so don't be too shocked when now and then your body seems to be screaming for a smoke. You are powerful enough to tell your body "no."

If you decide to go for sudden withdrawal, make a firm promise to yourself and then tell everyone who cares about you that you have done so. If your own self-respect is overshadowed by the craving, perhaps the opinions of others will help turn the tide. Throw out every cigarette you have. Ask your co-workers to refrain from smoking in your office. Set a date when you will smoke your last cigarette and stick to it. As the target date approaches, fill your time with enjoyable activities—preferably in places where smoking is prohibited.

Just how long the craving for cigarettes will last is an individual matter; it will eventually pass. Don't be too frightened of physical discomfort. The nervousness, sleep disturbances, weight gain, fatigue, and inability to concentrate are predictable. But they don't last forever, and they won't kill you. Smoking, on the other hand, will.

Many people fear tobacco withdrawal and try to stop gradually. Actually, say the experts, this is definitely the more difficult method.

There are many variations, but most involve systematic reduction of dosage—either by allowing progressively fewer cigarettes each day, or by progressively smoking less of each cigarette (which is not always easy).

Experts advise setting precise goals for yourself and programming rewards and punishments into your campaign. For example, if your goal the first week is to cut back by one full pack, reward yourself with theater tickets or a weekend in the country if you succeed. Punish yourself by not permitting yourself to play tennis or see a movie that week if you fail. Set your rules in advance and stick to them. Don't fall into the trap of thinking such contrivances childish—we reward and punish ourselves unknowingly all the time.

---

tips for slowing down

There are as many tips on how to stop as there are people who kicked the habit; everyone has his or her own secret. These include:

Keep postponing the first cigarette of the day for a longer and longer time.

When you crave a cigarette, don't light up for at least three minutes. During that time change your thought pattern or activity.

Increase your physical activity.

Have another smoker join you in your campaign; making a wager might help too.

Substitute a cup of tea or chewing gum at times when you usually break the pace with a cigarette.

Set rules for where you can and cannot smoke.

Carry only one cigarette with you when you leave home in the morning.

Keep a daily cigarette count. On a piece of paper, make four columns: time of day, activity, mood, and, in the last column, rate the need for the cigarette: (1) most important, (2) above average, (3) average, (4) below average, (5) least important (you would not have missed it). Wrap the paper around your pack of cigarettes, and make your entries each time you feel like smoking.

That last suggestion comes from a pamphlet entitled How to Really Quit Smoking, published by the Life Extension Institute. It includes a four-week, step-by-step program for quitting.

Whichever method you try—and the choice depends on you and your situation—the most important element in your battle against cigarettes is motivation. Choose your own incentive after giving serious thought to all the implications of smoking. Somewhere there is one that will stir your sense of purpose, whether it is health, pride, the cost of cigarettes, your children, or whatever.

smokers anonymous: the smokenders program

If you've tried to quit on your own without success, you might try SmokEnders. 30,000 people have taken this nine-week course, and the organization claims that only 6 of every 100 ever smoke again. During the first five weeks, you gradually cut back the number of cigarettes you smoke and learn to live without nicotine. One by one, you do away with those formerly indispensable butts—after breakfast, with coffee, over drinks, after lunch, and the last one at night. You quit completely after the fifth-week meeting, but must attend four more sessions for reinforcement. It costs between $100 and $150, depending on location. For information, write SmokEnders World, Phillipsburg, N.J. 08865, or call (201) 454-4357.

minimum approach to cutting down

If you don't want to spend the time or money—or simply don't have a strong enough inclination to quit cigarettes—there are ways at least to minimize the health hazards:

Choose a low-tar, low-nicotine brand.
Don't smoke cigarettes all the way down—you get most of the tar and nicotine in the last few puffs.
Take fewer drags on each cigarette.
Don't inhale deeply.
Smoke fewer cigarettes. Get into the habit of skipping them for certain periods of the day.
Use a special filter. These will not only reduce tars and nicotine, but will force you to take another step before lighting up. Aquafilter, at 10 for $1, is one effective type.

Once you find the proper motivation half the battle has been won. Now it becomes a matter of practicing a new, nonsmoking behavior pattern. Remember that quitting the cigarette habit is not going to take anything away from your life—it is going to add strength, health, pride, and lots of other good things.

the price of alcohol

Scientists at the Harvard School of Public Health estimated in 1974 that business and industry lose about $15 billion a year on alcohol-related problems. A problem drinker misses an average of 22 work days a year; his chances of incurring an accident are two to four times greater than the nondrinker's. Three times as many medical benefits are payed to alcoholics. One estimate puts the average loss to a company at one-fourth the drinker's annual salary.

Estimates of the number of "problem drinkers" in the United States range from nine to nineteen million. The number of people whose drinking has "created some problem for themselves or their families or friends or employers, or with the police," is about nine million, says the National Institute on Alcohol Abuse and Alcoholism (NIAAA). Alcoholics Anonymous thinks ten million is more accurate. The NIAAA estimates that 25 percent of employee alcoholics are white-collar workers, 30 percent are manual workers, and 45 percent are professionals or managers.

Alcoholism

"Alcoholism is a disease!," Alcoholics Anonymous emphatically states. Indeed, medical authorities try to treat alcoholism from the same medical perspective as they would diabetes or tuberculosis. But it is not yet known why one individual will become an alcoholic—while another can drink moderately high quantities for years without incurring the physical addiction that marks alcoholism. AA defines *alcoholic* as "any person whose indulgence in alcohol continuously or periodically results in behavior disruptive to normal relations with his or her work, family, or society."

For a long time the problem was naively chalked up to "moral weakness;" later it was thought to occur only among the anxiety-ridden and self-indulgent individuals who could not cope with life sober. Most recently it has become evident that physiological factors are involved, perhaps to a greater degree than ever suspected.

Alcoholics seem to have some biochemical susceptibility to alcohol. This may be genetically determined; children of alcoholic parents are about 50 percent more likely to become alcoholics than the offspring of nondrinkers. However, some argue that the home environment, not heredity, is responsible in those cases. Whatever its origins, the alcoholic is most likely a victim of his own physiology—much like an allergy, perhaps—compounded by the mental compulsion to drink. Not all heavy drinkers become addicted to alcohol. Many can drink in moderation, and stop at will. The alcoholic cannot. The physiological theory contends that mental/emotional difficulties are a *byproduct* of alcoholism, not the cause. In the end, proponents of the mental and physical theories may have to settle for a draw—both are certainly involved.

Excessive stress, of course, is a major factor: alcohol is one of the most common antistress devices known. But not only does the alcohol fail to remove the stressor, it tends to weaken the individual and render him even more vulnerable to stress. Thus, stress and alcohol form a vicious cycle. As an AA spokesman put it, "If you drink because you have a problem, you have two problems—your original problem and alcohol."

Treatment of Alcoholism

The hallmark of alcoholism is the inability to drink in moderation; it is an all-or-nothing proposition. Alcoholics cannot safely introduce alcohol into their systems. Once they do, they lose all control, and drunkenness inevitably follows. As of yet, there is no known treatment for this physiological susceptibility. All the successful interventions, such as Alcoholics Anonymous (whose record is unsurpassed), deal with the mental obsession. If this can be controlled, the critical first drink will not be taken; only then can the alcoholic lead a normal life.

The biggest problem involves getting the alcoholic to confront his addiction, which is complicated by the social stigma and misunderstanding attached to the disease. Alcoholics prefer to think of themselves as merely heavy social drinkers. They are usually convinced that they could drink moderately any time they choose to. They scoff at suggestions to cut down.

But cutting down will help only those who are capable of drinking in moderation. For true alcoholics, such exhortations are not only useless, but potentially destructive. It is imperative, councils AA, that the alcoholic understand his complete inability to drink in moderation. Some dispute that notion, maintaining that full rehabilitation would bring the person to the point where he can safely enjoy social drinking. But for decades, AA has found that alcoholics who attempt moderate drinking can do so only for a very short period. They inevitably end up over the barrel again.

In perhaps 90 percent of cases, alcoholism results in death or hospitalization before effective treatment can be applied. For those who join AA or other programs, it is usually some crisis at home or work, that provides the spur to get help. In all cases, they must clearly see the destructive effects alcohol is having and be able to overcome any initial loss of esteem that may come with such an admission.

Despite innumerable government-sponsored programs and scientific studies, Alcoholics Anonymous remains the most effective treatment modality available. Composed of recovered alcoholics, AA is self-supporting through members' contributions. It is not allied with any sect, denomination, political, or social organization. The only requirement for membership is the desire to stop drinking. For information on AA, write to P.O. Box 459, New York, N.Y. 10017.

self evaluation: are you an alcoholic?

AA suggests asking yourself these ten questions. If you have many "yes" answers, there is a good chance that you are an alcoholic. The disease may be in its initial stages, but it might become chronic. In some cases, the addiction will stabilize almost immediately, while in others the physical susceptibility is such that it might take months or years. But if the tendency is present, it is only a matter of time, unless abstention is achieved.

1. Do you lie about how much you drink?
2. Do you gulp your drinks and sneak extras?
3. Do you drink to relieve feelings of inadequacy?
4. Do you drink to escape worry and to dispel the blues?
5. Do you drink when overtired, to "brace up"?
6. Is drinking affecting your peace of mind?
7. Is drinking making your home life unhappy?
8. Do you sometimes drink alone? Do you black out?
9. Do you require a drink the next morning?
10. Do you lose time from work due to drinking?

In addition to these questions, put yourself to the critical test. Decide what a moderate consumption would be for you and try to stick to it. If you can't, it is a safe bet that you are an alcoholic. If you remotely suspect that is the case, act as if it were unequivocally true.

How to Enjoy Moderation

Even if you are not an alcoholic you may be drinking too much. Doctors feel that social drinking is probably harmless, perhaps even psychologically beneficial as a mild tranquilizer. "There is even evidence now that one or two cocktails a day will lessen the buildup of cholesterol in the blood," says Dr. Frederick J. Stare, a Harvard nutritionist. But the bounds of moderation are difficult to maintain.

Medically speaking, excessive drinking is a major health risk. It decreases mental alertness, coordination, and judgement—drinking causes nearly half of the nation's 80,000 annual traffic fatalities. Alcohol also lowers the body's resistance to infectious diseases such as pneumonia. "In an alcoholic stupor, secretions laden with bacteria may overwhelm our lung defenses," states a Life Extension Institute pamphlet. "Additionally, as alcohol attacks the liver cells, their ability to produce the antibodies against infections can be impaired. Many other vital functions of the liver can also become badly damaged by alcohol to the point that the body cannot survive."

Ultimately, destruction of the liver cells can result in cirrhosis. In this condition the liver cannot neutralize toxic materials. Nor can it produce the proteins necessary for maintaining normal circulation of body fluids or the antibodies needed to fight against disease.

Because alcohol is high in calories, drinking can result in markedly lowered appetite. As a result, the intake of essential nutrients falls far below what is necessary for good health. This accounts in large measure for the liver and heart problems associated with drinking. But it is not just a matter of skipped meals. According to medical authorities, a person can eat three square meals a day and still develop malnutrition if he drinks heavily.

---

how to enjoy moderation

Alcohol need not be a hazard. Keep your consumption on the moderate, healthy side by following these basic guidelines:

Eat wholesome food before drinking to slow the rate at which alcohol enters your blood.
Drink only in convivial friendly circumstances.
Drink only when you are in a good frame of mind, not when you are troubled.
Drink only when all of your daily obligations have been accomplished.
If before dinner, eat a full meal and don't plan to resume drinking after eating.
Avoid alcohol when suffering from physical pain or discomfort.
Do not drink with people you dislike.
Drink alcohol only when you have the desire for it, favoring nonalcoholic drinks at other times.

As any drinker knows, the psychological effects of alcohol can also be dangerous, once the initial euphoria and tranquility are exceeded. Barriers come tumbling down, and although freedom from inner restraint may be one attraction of alcohol, its abuses range from the relatively innocent slanders of the obnoxious drunk to wrecked careers and broken homes. Or worse: reportedly, alcohol is a contributing factor in 50 percent of all homicides and 25 percent of all suicides.

---

the drinkwatchers alternative

If you must attend lunches and meetings where cocktails are usually served, total abstinence from drink, to your thinking, may be more threatening than alcoholism. "Many executives feel giving up alcohol and being stigmatized as an alcoholic would be a real detriment to their business lives," says Richard Hull, a co-director of Drink-watchers, Inc.

Two Alcoholics Anonymous dropouts founded the nonprofit group for people who reject the alcoholic label and the abstinence required by AA.

Drinkwatchers get together in small, weekly meetings to explore individual solutions to each member's drinking problem. The only label you acquire on joining is "participant," and you learn how to cut down—or give the stuff up altogether, without losing the social contacts that go with drinking.

Meetings are now held in 57 cities in the United States, Canada, and Mexico. Write Drinkwatchers, P.O. Box 1062, Burlingame, Calif. 94010.

Drinking at Work

The cost of problem drinking has given rise to a growing number of corporate programs to curb alcoholism. The National Council on Alcoholism feels that employee programs are the most promising means of treatment. In 1970, U.S. companies were operating about 300 programs. By the end of 1975, the number had more than doubled. General Motors, the Norfolk and Western Railroad, and Control Data Corporation all conduct promising innovative programs for their employees.

It is not easy to assess the level of problem drinking within an organization. Most drinkers keep their problem secret, and supervisors are reluctant to jeopardize the individual's job or social acceptance. This reluctance also extends to physicians. A report in the *Psychiatric Annals* states:

> Careful studies have indicated that highly motivated, intelligent physicians tend not to make the diagnosis of alcoholism in patients who are clearly suffering serious alcohol problems if the patient (1) is married, (2) voluntarily comes to an admitting service, (3) has another medical problem on which the physician can focus, (4) is gainfully employed, or (5) has health insurance. In other words, the tendency among physicians is to define alcoholism only among derelict people.

Early recognition is a vital factor in heading off disaster. Experts feel that employees and co-workers have a good advantage in identifying and helping problem drinkers. First, they can spot the problem at an early stage; drinking will invariably begin to affect the person's work performance. The second advantage involves "constructive coercion": the threat of getting fired is a common fear among drinkers, and will often supply sufficient motivation even when other considerations cannot.

Traditionally, industry programs revolved around spotting alcoholics by readily observable signs—bloodshot eyes, trembling, or alcoholic breath. More recently, referrals to alcoholism programs have been based on unsatisfactory performance, rule violations, and other observable signs of deterioration. The approach favored by the National Council on Alcoholism is to refer the individual to a general counseling service whenever performance drops below standards and ordinary methods do not work. This places both diagnosis and decisions regarding treatment in qualified hands.

---

corporate alcoholism programs

These are the factors generally considered important for a successful employee alcoholism program:

State the policy clearly.
Inform employees and supervisors that the policy will be uniformly enforced.
Encourage problem drinkers to seek treatment without fear of immediate dismissal.
Guarantee confidentiality.
Recognize alcoholism as an illness and the drinker as a patient who needs help.
Provide machinery for obtaining professional treatment and outside referrals.
Include some degree of "constructive coercion," such as the threat of discharge if treatment fails to improve performance.
Locate the counseling unit away from other departments to assure privacy.
Train supervisors to evaluate job performance.
Include hospital care for alcoholism in insurance coverage.

Experts also feel that in-house programs should not attempt to disguise the fact that their target is alcoholism through the use of a sanitized euphemism like "troubled employee program." They advocate recognizing alcoholism as such, and treating it as an illness that can be overcome.

---

for further information on alcoholism:

Corporate Headquarters Alcoholism Project
120 E. 56th Street, Suite 240
New York, N.Y. 10022

National Clearinghouse for Alcohol Information
NIAAA
P.O. Box 2345
Rockville, Maryland 20852

National Council on Alcoholism
733 Third Avenue
New York, N.Y. 10017

Your local chapter of Alcoholics Anonymous

See *Drinking on the Job,* a publication of the Public Affairs Committee, 381 Park Avenue South, New York, N.Y. 10016.

drugs on the job

The Drug Abuse Warning Network (DAWN), is a computerized data service that provides the government with monthly reports on which drugs have propelled users into hospital emergency rooms or morgues. A recent report showed that Valium, a commonly used tranquilizer, caused more emergency-room complications than any other drug. Barbiturates were the biggest killer, and the most lethal combination was Valium and alcohol.

DAWN's list of the ten most dangerous drugs as reported in *The Village Voice,* shows that virtually all of them are commonly prescribed or regularly purchased over the counter:

1. Valium
2. alcohol in combination with other drugs
3. heroin and other morphine derivatives
4. aspirin
5. flurazapam (a tranquilizer)
6. Darvon
7. Librium
8. Elavil
9. phenobarbitol
10. secobarbital

Popping pills unfortunately has become a way of life for many executives, some of whom rely quite heavily on tranquilizers to get them through difficult days, and on amphetamines (pep pills) to zip them up when fatigue (or the tranquilizers) overtakes them. Pill taking represents a major health menace, particularly when done by a drinker. Pills are definitely not the answer to stress.

stimulants and depressants

	Description	Effects	How To Spot Abuser	Dangers
Amphetamine	Central nervous system stimulant, often prescribed for reducing appetite or to increase energy.	Increases alertness, reduces tiredness, increases energy, relieves depression.	Abnormal cheerfulness, unusual amount of energy, tendency to talk excessively about anything; jumpy, irritable, hyperactive; perhaps paranoia and hallucinations.	High blood pressure, abnormal heart rhythms, irrational behavior, weight loss, aggressiveness, extreme nervousness, hallucinations, psychic dependence.
Barbiturates	Barbiturate acid derivatives used as sedatives or hypnotics. Act as depressant to central nervous system.	Calming, tranquilizing effect; in small amounts, produces light-heartedness; sedation and narcosis.	Appearance of drunkenness without smell of alcohol; sluggish; gloomy; thick speech; staggering and incoordination; quarrelsome.	Coma and death due to respiratory failure; overdose can be fatal; combination with alcohol especially dangerous; physical and psychic addiction from which withdrawl is extremely difficult.

current drug usage profile

The following table is derived from a study conducted by the Division of Research of the New York State Narcotic Addiction Control Commission. The sample consisted of 1,692,000 professionals, technical workers, managers, and owners of businesses.

Drug	Never Used	Infrequent Users (1–5 times per month)	Regular Users (At least 6 times per month)	Percent of Regular Users Who Used Drug at Work
Marijuana	86.8%	3.8%	2.8%	20.8%
Heroin	96.7		.2	
LSD	96.0	0.7	0.1	50.0
Methedrine	96.2	0.3	0.1	50.0
Barbiturates	74.1	4.0	2.6	11.4
Nonbarbiturate sedative/hypnotic	86.0	3 1	1.2	
Relaxants	74.3	6.7	3.0	36.0
Major tranquilizers	93.0	1.0	0.2	
Antidepressants	95.3	1.2		
Pep Pills	89.2	2.2	0.8	28.6
Diet Pills	86.8	1.4	2.0	11.8
Narcotics (not heroin)	84.6	1.2	0.2	75.0

The statistics in the table above were gathered in 1971. There is every reason to believe that drug usage has risen since then. While the percentages may not seem high, they add up to a lot of drug use in any given company. This is especially true when the figures for other occupational groups are included. Clerical and other white-collar workers, for example, used major tranquilizers four times as often as the managerial/professional group did. As a nation, we use three billion doses of tranquilizers and barbiturates a year.

Virtually every medical authority will say the same thing about mood-altering drugs: they do not solve any problems, they merely cover them up temporarily, while making things worse in the end.

how specific stress disorders are treated

If prevention has failed—or was never attempted—certain well-known stress disorders tend to appear, including atherosclerosis, hypertension, ulcers, and headaches. We have discussed how these problems are detected in chapter three. Here is a review of the steps medical science can take to deal with them.

Atherosclerosis

When serious coronary artery blockage is discovered, the treatment typically used in severe cases is bypass surgery—commonly a saphenous-vein bypass. A leg vein is used to bypass the blockage. For this the heart must be temporarily stopped, and an artificial pump is used during the operation. The substitute artery is grafted in place to circumvent the clogged vessel.

Surgery is a radical and risky procedure. The medical community is polarized on how advisable it is, and whether or not there are reasonable alternatives to the estimated 70,000 surgeries performed each year. In a first-rate, major hospital the mortality rate from such surgery is four to five percent. In a few leading centers specializing in heart surgery, the mortality rate is said to be as low as one or two percent. (Proponents point out, however, that patients requiring surgery will be high risks under any conditions.)

Leading heart surgeon Michael De Bakey defends the bypass, citing data showing that 92 percent of patients "are living as long as their counterparts in the general population." A Wall Street insurance executive whose coronary-bypass surgery corrected two blockages notes that his recovery was far easier than he had expected. "I had few restraints put on my activity once I returned home," he says. "I started reading novels and getting about the house quite nicely. In a few weeks I was back at the office, and in two months' time I started tennis."

With bypass surgery, typical angina pains are generally eliminated, and the patient's range of activities is substantially increased. As yet, there is no evidence that surgery can lengthen life span, but some feel that surgery will be shown to lengthen lives.

leading centers for heart surgery

City	Name of Center
Boston	Peter Bent Brigham Hospital
Cleveland	Cleveland Clinic
Houston	Methodist Hospital
Milwaukee	St. Joseph's Hospital
New York	New York University Medical Center
Palo Alto, Calif.	Stanford University Medical Center

But not everyone is satisfied with bypass surgery, despite its good track record. Losing between one and five of every 100 patients may seem low, but some consider it too high. Reportedly, two studies indicate that 20 to 30 percent of the grafts performed during bypass surgery become occluded within a year.

Nathan Pritikin, director of the Longevity Institute and a staunch opponent of surgery, claims that "the insertion of vein grafts causes acceleration of disease in the arteries receiving the grafts. The insertion of grafts increases the likelihood that new total occlusions will develop in the arteries at points both before and after the graft insertion site."

According to opponents of surgery, the heart is capable of establishing its own bypasses unless there has been a massive blockage of a major artery. In addition, many claim that diet and exercise can promote the conditions whereby the body will not only create its own bypasses, but eliminate arterial plaques as well.

The debate is unlikely to subside; ultimately, it is a matter for patient and physician to decide. With or without surgery, however, it is clear that heart patients (or anyone concerned with his or her heart) must be prepared to make changes in habits: restricting fatty foods, cutting down alcohol consumption, moderating the amount of workaday tension, and, perhaps most important, eliminating tobacco (some cardiologists refuse to continue treating coronary patients who insist upon smoking). The responsibility is yours. Cardiologists Meyer Friedman and Ray Rosenman state emphatically: "We know of no other disease whose outcome depends so little upon what is done *for* the patient and so much upon what is done *by* the patient."

how to help a heart-attack victim

There is nothing quite so frightening as being present when a friend or colleague suffers a heart attack. The cardinal rule: act without a minute's delay. The first symptom is usually a prolonged pain in the center of the chest behind the breast bone. It can be mild or severe and may spread into the arm, back, neck, or jaw.

If the person merely has chest pains and feels shaky, first quickly discourage him from insisting that it is only "indigestion"—a fearful denial of reality among some—and get him to a hospital fast.

Do not wait for the 10 or 15 minutes it might take for an ambulance to arrive.

If the attack is obvious, and if the victim is unconscious but breathing, take him quickly to a hospital without attempting any form of first aid.

If the victim is unconscious and not breathing, start emergency aid immediately. Brain damage occurs within four to six minutes after blood stops flowing. Apply cardiopulmonary resuscitation (CPR):

Put the victim on his back. Lift his neck with one hand, and push gently down on his forehead with the other. This allows free breathing.

If there is still no breath, pinch the victim's nose shut, breathe deeply, and administer four deep breaths into the victim's mouth.

Check the victim's pulse, using the carotid artery that is in a groove behind the voice box. If there is no pulse, you will need to start artificial circulation.

Compress the heart muscle externally to force it into action. Put the heel of your hand 1 in. to 1 1/2 in. above the lower tip of the breastbone and your other hand on top. Compress the breastbone (of an adult) about 1 1/2 in. to 2 in., using a rhythmic, rocking motion. Do about 80 chest compressions per minute.

Remember that this is lifesaving, emergency action and that although the victim might be injured by your efforts, the alternative—when there is no heartbeat and no breath—is death. A local office of the American Heart Association will furnish further details and information. Note also that CPR requires practice.

Hypertension

According to Dr. Paul N. Yu, former president of the American Heart Association, "Over 80 percent of patients are successfully treated with drugs." In most cases daily doses may be a lifelong requirement, but apparently it is worth the effort, particularly in severe cases. The death rate in patients whose blood pressure is medically controlled has been reduced, as have symptoms of heart disease, kidney disorders, and strokes related to hypertension.

The antihypertensive drugs are expensive, and most produce side effects of one kind or another:

dizziness
dry mouth
skin rashes
nasal congestion
loss of potassium
tiredness

Some side effects are not noticeable, but will show up in blood tests. Have your doctor monitor your blood and adjust the dosage accordingly.

There are hundreds of varieties of antihypertensive drugs, none of which is universally effective or equally well tolerated by patients

They fall into three general categories: drugs that block the nerve impulses to blood vessels, those that eliminate extra bodily fluids, and those that directly relax blood vessels.

---

widely used antihypertension drugs

Diuretics These eliminate excess salts and fluids from the body. Some researchers feel that the excretion of sodium may have a relaxing effect on the arterioles, the small branches of the arterial system that feed the capillaries. Diuretics are sometimes used alone, and sometimes in combination with other medication.

Alphamethyldopa This works by inhibiting the activity of the sympathetic nervous system, and is said to be effective for approximately half of all hypertensive patients.

Guanethidine This inhibits the release of norepinephrine, the adrenal hormone that stimulates heart rate. This drug is extremely potent, and is used mainly in the treatment of sustained and accelerating hypertension.

Hydralazine Usually used in combination with a diuretic or a sympathetic nervous system depressant, this drug works by relaxing the smooth muscles of the arterioles, thus dilating them.

For some people with high blood pressure a modification in lifestyle could be sufficient: allow for greater rest and relaxation (Transcendental Meditation has been found to normalize blood pressure), moderation in diet (cutting down salt and fat intake), regular but moderate exercise. Above all, have your blood pressure checked regularly. Many large corporations have mobile units to check executive's blood pressure right at their desks.

Ulcers

Most of us know at least one person who is on a bland diet because of ulcers: strained, unseasoned foods, and regular doses of milk. The purpose of this is to keep the gastric juices from attacking the stomach lining. Recently, however, the restrictive diet has lost favor.

Two decades ago, Dr. Stewart Wolf discovered that the lining of the stomach and duodenum can tolerate more irritation than the skin. Substances that are not abrasive to the skin will not damage internal organ linings either; the damage is done by acids and enzymes produced by the body itself.

The latest opinion on the use of diet for ulcer patients is expressed by Dr. Arthur Schwabe, a gastroenterologist: "Patients should be encouraged to eat three nutritious, enjoyable meals of their own choosing every day."

What about other treatments? At a 1976 conference that examined every traditional ulcer treatment, virtually all were refuted. Antacids, on which $100 million is spent annually, were a chief target. Dr. Schwabe is in favor of tailoring the safer antacids to the individual's needs, a practice that is rarely followed. Medications containing calcium should not be used, he feels, and patients with high blood pressure should avoid medicines that contain a high percentage of sodium. Liquid antacids are preferred over tablets.

Many physicians believe that antacids are no better than placebos, partially because the frequency with which they must be taken makes it difficult for patients to comply with doctor's orders. One study found that 78 percent of patients using antacids had their ulcers healed, but so did 45 percent who had taken placebos. More significantly, according to Gilbert Cant in the *New York Times;* "The patients whose ulcers had healed did not *feel* any better than those with unhealed craters remaining. The two groups complained with equal vehemence of continuing, painful symptoms."

Antispasmodic drugs have also been used in ulcer treatment, to the tune of $65 million a year. But they can lead to such side effects as blurred vision, constipation, and urinary retention.

If an ulcer is bleeding into the intestine, or it results in a perforated stomach or duodenal wall, surgery is virtually compulsory. Avoid it otherwise. Reportedly, 10 to 20 percent of all surgery patients suffer relapses. Postoperative handicaps include possible diarrhea and nausea, restrictions on diet and alcohol consumption, and continual gulping of antacids.

The most promising feature in an otherwise bleak landscape for ulcer sufferers is a radically new medication. Certain receptor cells found in the lower stomach wall provoke the secretion of excess acid when stimulated by histamine. After many trials, Professor James W. Black of London's University College developed *cimetidine,* an antihistamine that blocks the interraction of histamine with these receptor cells. The F.D.A. recently gave limited approval for its use.

Ulcers remain a mystery. Available treatments are either viewed skeptically, have harmful side effects, or are brand new and relatively untested. The outlook is positive in the medical community, however, where researchers are confident that new discoveries such as cimetidine will eventually replace less effective medication and surgery. In the meantime, a change in life-style to keep stress under control is the best way to prevent and treat ulcers. Take it easy, say the experts. There are better ways to show that you are a hard-working, upward-striving, and conscientious executive than to wear a peptic ulcer as a merit badge.

Diabetes

"When patients find out that they have diabetes," warns Dr. Joseph Skon, former president of an affiliate of the American Diabetes Association, "they feel frustration, depression, and a sense of being less than human."

If you are diagnosed diabetic, it by no means spells the end of your career, or a lifetime of suffering.

In many cases, careful attention to diet, weight, exercise, and other factors prescribed by your doctor can help limit the consequences of the disease. In some cases, however, patients require regular insulin injections. Contact your local chapter of the ADA for a doctor who is expert in treating diabetes. With the help of a trained dietician, the doctor will work out the best regiment for you.

Once treatment begins, you should be able to live and work pretty much as you always have. Bernard A. Malm, 65-year-old chairman of DeSoto, Inc. in Des Plaines, Illinois, has been a diabetic for thirty years. "The first thing to do," he says, "is admit to yourself that you have the disease. Then, with special care and training you'll do very well. Most important, decide that you are going to work with it."

You can still keep up with your favorite sport. Charles Schreiber, an account executive at N. W. Ayer ABH International New York, is 46 and has had diabetes for five years. Insulin is part of his daily routine, and missing a mealtime could lead to a hypoglycemic (low blood sugar) reaction. But Schreiber hasn't given up his favorite sport, sailing. "I take along a do-it-yourself dextrose kit," says Schreiber, "and a supply of peanut butter for instant energy."

Above all, if you are a diabetic, don't keep it a secret. Tell your employer and carry a Medic Alert emblem and wallet card with detailed information on your medical history. The emblem, in bracelet or necklace form, can be obtained for a lifetime fee of $7 from the International Medic Alert Foundation, P.O. Box 1009, Turlock, Calif., 95380, or from one of its offices in your area.

Headaches

Drugs have been the primary treatment modality until quite recently, when they became suspect. Aspirin, of course, has been used to dull pain. Its side effects are known to be risky. For migraine, a combination of caffeine and ergotamine tartrate is often used to constrict the expanded blood vessels. A more powerful drug was discovered in the 1960s. Called *methylsergide maleate,* or Sansert, this chemical relation to LSD must be used with extreme caution because its side effects include hallucinations, nausea, and vascular disease.

Drugs, however, can only diminish symptoms; they do not touch the underlying cause. Recently, non-drug therapies have been employed with varying degrees of success. Most seem to work for some migraine sufferers some of the time.

Dr. John B. Brainard advocates changes in diet and life-style: reduce salt intake; avoid smoke-filled rooms; shun alcohol; avoid ripened cheese, chocolate, nuts, and ham; get plenty of rest.

Dr. Seymour Diamond and others have reported considerable success treating migraines with biofeedback (see chapter eight). He trains patients to raise the temperature in their hands, which increases the amount of blood flow to that area while, presumably, reducing it in the head.

Dr. Diamond's findings have been verified by other researchers, including some of the Menninger Clinic and the Mayo Clinic. Dr. Charles Stroebel of Hartford's Institute of Living reports that 70 to 80 percent of his patients obtained relief from migraines through biofeedback.

---

headache program at ehe

The StressControl Center at Executive Health Examiners has incorporated biofeedback techniques into a medically supervised training program. Registered nurses, specially trained in relaxation techniques, provide private sessions, promised to give "significant relief from muscle tension headaches and vascular tension headaches." The program lasts about five weeks; sessions last 1 to 1 1/2 hours per week; the cost is $215 per person.

Be leary of drugs, and be especially leary of any "headache clinic" that promises miracle cures for headaches through the use of medication. "Overuse of pain pills is one of the great American problems," says Dr. Donald J. Dalessio, head of the neurology division at Scripps Clinic and Research Foundation in La Jolla, California. "Patients with chronic headaches should be told that they can't be cured but frequently can be helped, and that their headaches probably won't kill them, but the medications may."

defense strategies for life

Holistic health requires a holistic view of life. No longer is it reasonable to isolate symptoms and treatments, habits and life-styles, foods and drugs from the state of well-being of the *whole* person. The best way to maximize your own health comes from an intelligent balance of common sense and medical experience. The essence of this technique is to take as active an interest in the efficiency of body and mind as you would in any large vital investment or project.

Be alert to what agrees with you, and especially to what interferes with your best performance. Foster the former and minimize the latter. Stay as aware as you can of how you are doing in life. Real success includes real health.

Two major approaches have evolved to combat disease—treatment and prevention. Obviously, prevention is preferable, if the immediate investment of time and effort is not too great (for some, the joy of smoking seems to outweigh the tragedy it will probably bring). But in both cases, stress is the common foe, and its archenemies are rest, regularity, and moderation.

The next five chapters apply this holistic style of thinking to both offense and defense in the main areas of life accessible to us: behavior and attitudes (chapter five), exercise (chapter six), diet (chapter seven), mental techniques (chapter eight), and the body *and* the mind's most basic resource—a good night's sleep (chapter nine).

————— recommended reading: chapter 4 —————

Control of Migraine, John B. Brainard (New York: Norton, 1977).

Employee Drug Abuse, Chambers and Heckman (Boston: Cahners, 1972).

"Heart Disease: New Ways to Reduce the Risk," *Business Week,* October 10, 1977.

How To Be Your Own Doctor (Sometimes), Keith W. Sehnert (New York: Grossett & Dunlap, 1976).

How to Control Your Drinking, William Miller and Ricardo Munoz (Englewood Cliffs, N.J.: Prentice-Hall, 1976).

How to Stop Smoking, Herbert Brean (New York: Pocket Books, 1975).

Our Bodies, Our Selves, Boston Women's Health Book Collective (New York: Simon & Schuster, 1976).

Quick Headache Relief Without Drugs, Howard Kurland (New York: Morrow, 1977).

Symptoms: The Complete Home Medical Encyclopedia, Sigmund Miller (New York: Crowell, 1977).

Take Care of Yourself: A Consumer's Guide to Medical Care, Donald Vickery and James Fries, (Reading, Mass.: Addison-Wesley, 1976).

Talk Back to Your Doctor: How to Demand (And Recognize) High Quality Health Care, Arthur Levin (New York: Doubleday, 1975).

The People's Pharmacy, Joe Graedon (New York: St. Martin's Press, 1976).

Why Drinking Can be Good for You, Morris Chafetz (Briarcliff Manor, N.Y.: Stein & Day, 1976).

the psychological dimension

The greatest mistake in the treatment of diseases is that there are physicians for the body and physicians for the soul, although the two cannot be separated.——Plato

mind and body

The most important aspect of holistic health is the understanding that mind and body are a "cooperative unit": what affects one will affect the other, and a person is a whole that far exceeds the limitations of component parts. It is obvious that physical malfunctions can drastically interfere with mental performance, but the realization that mental and emotional states can materially contribute to physical disease is new to Western medicine. It finally has hit home: medical authorities now acknowledge that the nonphysical dimension is an essential element in preventing and treating most illnesses.

For decades, the connection between emotional stress and minor visceral problems like upset stomach as been well known. More recently, a strong relationship between behavior and the killer diseases, particularly cardiovascular illness, has also been substantiated. Dr. C. David Jenkins, reviewing the literature for the New England Journal of Medicine (April 29 and May 6, 1976) concludes: "The behavioral risk factor made an independent contribution to coronary risk after the influences of the standard biologic risk factors ... were accounted for statistically."

The fight-or-flight response, repeatedly fired off by worry, emotional upset, fear, pressing deadlines, and other threatening situations, will interfere with the nervous system and wear down the body. The

self-evaluation: the glazer-stresscontrol life-style questionnaire*

As you can see, each scale below is composed of a pair of adjectives or phrases separated by a series of horizontal lines. Each pair has been chosen to represent two kinds of contrasting behavior. Each of us belongs somewhere along the line between the two extremes. Since most of us are neither the most competitive nor the least competitive person we know, put a check mark where you think you belong between the two extremes.

		1	2	3	4	5	6	7	
1.	Doesn't mind leaving things temporarily unfinished	—	—	—	—	—	—	—	Must get things finished once started
2.	Calm and unhurried about appointments	—	—	—	—	—	—	—	Never late for appointments
3.	Not competitive	—	—	—	—	—	—	—	Highly competitive
4.	Listens well, lets others finish speaking	—	—	—	—	—	—	—	Anticipates others in conversation (nods, interrupts, finishes sentences for the other)
5.	Never in a hurry, even when pressured	—	—	—	—	—	—	—	Always in a hurry
6.	Able to wait calmly	—	—	—	—	—	—	—	Uneasy when waiting
7.	Easygoing	—	—	—	—	—	—	—	Always going full speed ahead

Continued on following page.

		1	2	3	4	5	6	7	
8.	Takes one thing at a time	—	—	—	—	—	—	—	Tries to do more than one thing at a time, thinks about what to do next
9.	Slow and deliberate in speech	—	—	—	—	—	—	—	Vigorous and forceful in speech (uses a lot of gestures)
10.	Concerned with satisfying himself, not others	—	—	—	—	—	—	—	Wants recognition by others for a job well done
11.	Slow doing things	—	—	—	—	—	—	—	Fast doing things (eating, walking, etc.)
12.	Easygoing	—	—	—	—	—	—	—	Hard driving
13.	Expresses feelings openly	—	—	—	—	—	—	—	Holds feelings in
14.	Has a large number of interests	—	—	—	—	—	—	—	Few interests outside work
15.	Satisfied with job	—	—	—	—	—	—	—	Ambitious, wants quick advancement on job
16.	Never sets own deadlines	—	—	—	—	—	—	—	Often sets own deadlines
17.	Feels limited responsibility	—	—	—	—	—	—	—	Always feels responsible
18.	Never judges things in terms of numbers	—	—	—	—	—	—	—	Often judges performance in terms of numbers (how many, how much)
19.	Casual about work	—	—	—	—	—	—	—	Takes work very seriously (works weekends, brings work home)
20.	Not very precise	—	—	—	—	—	—	—	Very precise (careful about detail)

SCORING: Assign a value from 1 to 7 for each score. Total them up. The categories are as follows:

Total score = 110–140: Type A$_1$.

If you are in this category, and especially if you are over 40 and smoke, you are likely to have a high risk of developing cardiac illness.

Continued on following page.

self-evaluation: the glazer-stresscontrol life-style questionnaire*

Total score = 80–109: Type A₂.

You are in the direction of being cardiac prone, but your risk is not as high as the A₁. You should, nevertheless, pay careful attention to the advice given to all Type A's.

Total score = 60–79: Type AB..

You are an admixture of A and B patterns. This is a healthier pattern than either A₁ or A₂, but you have the potential for slipping into A behavior and you should recognize this.

Total score = 30–59: Type B₂.

Your behavior is on the less-cardiac-prone end of the spectrum. You are generally relaxed and cope adequately with stress.

Total score = 0–29: Type B₁.

You tend to the extreme of non-cardiac traits. Your behavior expresses few of the reactions associated with cardiac disease.

This test will give you some idea of where you stand in the discussion of Type A behavior that follows. The higher your score, the more cardiac prone you tend to be. Remember, though, even B persons occasionally slip into A behavior, and any of these patterns can change over time.

*This questionnaire was designed for this book by Dr. Howard I. Glazer, director of behavior management systems at EHE Stresscontrol Systems, Inc.

more intense the stress, the weaker the system, and—in the familiar vicious cycle—the more vulnerable to further emotional strain. A wide variety of mental or physical breakdowns can result.

Besides serious illness, there are other consequences of mental and emotional problems, and they all cost money. Interpersonal friction, accidents (85 percent of industrial accidents are said to be stress induced), absenteeism, and poor performance are all expensive. According to the National Association for Mental Health, one employee with emotional problems costs his organization $1622 per year, with a total annual loss in productivity to U.S. business of $17 billion.

Psychology and Management

Executives are now recognizing the need to manage emotions that can damage their health and their work. In most cases it is informal—a trusted physician or peer to whom the executive can open up provides emotional support and learned advice. In other instances, professional counseling may be required.

"Without question," says Dr. Sidney Lecker, director of EHE's StressControl Systems, Inc., "there's a trend toward the use of mental health professionals by business." Lecker lauds the trend, but feels it is moving too slowly. "We're trying to make companies aware of the need to consider the psychological milieu a person is placed in," he says.

Lecker feels that psychologists should not only deal with troubled persons, but work on the organizational level as well. He would like to see organizational case studies, which would identify sources of stress and apply remedies to suit the character of the company.

As *Newsweek* observes, the situation is "a startling turnaround from the days when a worker who let it be known that he was seeing a psychiatrist might well be jeopardizing his career." An estimated 500 psychiatrists and psychologists are now employed by such corporate giants as General Motors, U.S. Steel, and I.B.M. But while mental and emotional problems have come well out of the closet, there is still some stigma attached to seeing a psychologist.

Says a leading New York psychiatrist, "The problem is to get the businessman to relax—and forget his scruples about talking with a 'shrink.'" Examing physicians maintain that the more an executive opens up, the greater the chances of recognizing precursors of illness such as job worry, irritability, excessive drinking, or hostility. But for management professionals, resistance to psychiatric input may not be easy to overcome. Says Dr. Herbert Klemme of the Menninger Clinic in Topeka, Kansas, "The very qualities that make an executive successful—independence and drive—often prevent him from seeking the kind of help he needs."

Self-Esteem vs. Self-Preservation

There should be no stigma attached to consulting a mental health expert. Ordinary emotional problems are not pathological; the executive under stress is not mentally ill. The "famous" severe mental illnesses—schizophrenia, manic-depressive psychosis, and so on—are rarely found in executive suites, or at any other level of management.

Nor should consultation await serious breakdowns. With the world as complex as it is, and with sources of stress so ubiquitous, it is becoming more and more evident that executives can benefit a good deal from the expertise of those who have studied human behavior. Like physicians, mental health experts are now directing their skills toward prevention. It is, after all, the way we *respond* to stress, not so much the stressors themselves, that determines whether or not the impact will be large or small.

———————— the type a behavior pattern ————————

About 25 years ago, San Francisco cardiologists Meyer Friedman and Ray Rosenman began investigating the connection between behavior and heart disease. Informal observations and surveys had led them to suspect that the effects of competition and job deadlines were more insidious than previously imagined. When they discovered that the blood cholesterol levels of accountants peaked at tax time, Friedman and Rosenman embarked on a massive study to determine which personality and behavior variables most influenced the likelihood of heart disease. Their work lasted for ten years (1960–1970), and involved 35,000 men aged 31–59, each of whom were given a behavioral classification based on interviews and observations. None had any record of heart disease. By 1970, 257 had developed coronary heart disease—70 percent of the victims were what the cardiologists had categorized as Type A.

Type A Defined

Friedman and Rosenman call it "an action-emotion complex that can be observed in any person who is *aggressively* involved in a *chronic, incessant* struggle to achieve more and more in less and less time, and if required to do so, against the opposing efforts of other things or other persons."

By contrast, the Type B is "rarely harried by desires to obtain a wildly increasing number of things or participate in an endlessly growing series of events in an ever decreasing amount of time."

---

main characteristics of the type a individual

Sense of Time Urgency They have "hurry sickness," always trying to stuff more into less time. They create deadlines if none exist and substitute the quick for the better. (B's find time to ponder, weigh alternatives, experiment; they feel there is plenty of time.)

Quest for Numbers Numbers—of dollars, of achievements, or other quantifiable items, are indices of prowess and achievement to the Type A. B's are more quality than quantity oriented.

Insecurity of Status A's are outwardly confident and self-assured, but are often insecure underneath. They are constantly struggling for recognition through numbers of achievements. They do not measure themselves by present status, but by the rate at which it improves.

Aggression and Hostility A's are extremely competitive. They tend to always challenge other people—in sports, games, work, or even discussions. Their free-floating hostility is not easily detected, but there is often a note of rancor in their speech. They might fume at something a B will pass right over or laugh at.

Ironically, many Type A's persist in their pattern because they think it is necessary for the accomplishment of their goals. But most astute observers feel that the higher rungs of achievement are occupied by as many Type B's, if not more.

"The Type A's are not always successful businessmen," adds Dr. Howard Glazer. "They can be successful on a managerial level, even a high executive level, but when it comes to making selections and priorities, Type A's do not do well."

Why Type A's get Heart Attacks

Friedman and Rosenman concluded that "in the absence of Type A Behavior Pattern, coronary heart disease almost never occurs before 70 years of age, regardless of the fatty foods eaten, the cigarettes smoked, or the lack of exercise. But when this behavior pattern is present, coronary heart disease can easily erupt in one's 30s or 40s."

Interestingly, the physicians found that Type A's were not only three times as likely to develop heart disease than Type B's, but that A's who were low on other risk factors were still more cardiac prone than B's who smoked, were hypertensive, and whose family histories included heart attacks.

Type A behavior, Friedman and Rosenman claim, leads to an excess discharge of the so-called stress hormones—cortisol, epinephrine, and norepinephrine. Type A's have an excess of insulin in their blood and take three to four times longer to rid their body of dietary cholesterol after each meal. These changes, they explain, can lead to the narrowing of blood vessels and increased deposits of clotting elements in the blood.

But other experts feel that Freidman and Rosenman underplay the importance of standard risk factors. Said one opponent: "They've in effect told the American public that they could smoke what they want, drink what they want, eat what they want, and it doesn't make a difference. If you're Type A, that's what's going to do it to you." Some feel that stress-related behavior can harm only an already damaged cardiovascular system, and that improper habits will cause heart attacks regardless of personality.

Friedman and Rosenman are aware that research to date has only uncovered a *correlation* between Type A behavior and heart disease. It has not established that Type A behavior *causes* heart disease—or that a change in behavior patterns can *prevent* attacks. But one thing is clear: Type A behavior is a definite risk factor.

Type A individuals are especially likely to score high in other risk factors. "As a group," write Friedman and Rosenman, "most Type A subjects show a higher serum cholesterol, a higher serum fat, more diabetic-like traits or precursors, smoke more cigarettes, excercise less (because they can't find time to do so), are 'overdriving' certain of their endocrine glands, ... eat meals rich in cholesterol and animal fat, and also suffer more from high blood pressure than Type B subjects."

We may therefore be dealing with chickens and eggs. But when so many factors are involved, the best thing to do is take charge of all of them. And that must, no doubt, include our own behavior, despite the Type A tendency to look for quick, nonthreatening solutions. Changing behavior involves a certain amount of introspection that (here's Catch-22 again) most Type A's are reluctant to undergo.

How to Identify a Type A

Obviously, few of us are unequivocal A's or B's. Most of us exhibit a blend of both characteristics. The following questionnaire will help you assess yourself. Even a cursory examination of the behavior patterns associated with Type A's should be enough to afford a good idea of your own category. Friedman and Rosenman suggest also checking with a friend or spouse to see what they think. If friends disagree with you, they say, the other person is probably right.

detecting the type a behavior pattern

Vocal Explosiveness Do you overemphasize key words in ordinary speech and speed up the last few words of a sentence?

Constant Motion Do you move, walk, and eat rapidly?

Impatience Do you find yourself hurrying the speech of others or finishing their sentences for them? Is it anguish to wait on line? Do you always rush your reading? Do slow drivers in your lane make you boil?

Thinking or Doing Two or More Things at Once Do you dictate letters while driving? Do you use an electric razor while reading or eating?

Dominating Conversation Do you always change the topic to subjects that interest you? Is it difficult to restrain from cutting in? When you can't cut in, do you pretend to listen while thinking of something else?

Feeling Guilty When Relaxing Do you begin to lose respect for yourself when you do nothing for a few hours? Do you have few hobbies or diversions outside work? Do you consider noncompetitive physical activities a waste of time?

Preoccupation with Having, Not Being Do you fail to find time to improve yourself or explore new and interesting things? Have you neglected the aesthetic side of life for the sake of accumulating achievements?

Scheduling More and More in Less and Less Time Do you fail to make allowances for unforseen contingencies? Do you always feel pressured by time? Do you create deadlines if none exist?

Feeling Compelled to Challenge Others Do you find yourself competing even when the situation doesn't require it? (They say that nothing arouses the aggressive hostility of a Type A more than another Type A.)

Nervous Tics or Gestures Do you frequently clench your fist, bang your hand on the table, or pound your fist into your palm to drive home a point? Do you habitually clench your jaw or grind your teeth?

Fear of Slowing Down Do you feel that your success is due to your ability to do things faster than others?

Attachment to the Numbers Game Do you find yourself committed to translating achievement in terms of quantity instead of quality?

What to Do about Type A Behavior

Dr. Friedman claims that, subsequent to his own heart attack, he took stock of himself in the manner he recommends to other Type A's (see box above). A prototypical Type A himself, he decided to adopt a Type

B pattern, even wearing old tweedy sports coats. He moved his family to a quiet suburb. He avoided cocktail parties, gave up his membership on every committee except one, and read books he couldn't rush through. "I take time to daydream now," he says. "At lunchtime I go into St. Mary's Cathedral and look at the stained glass windows." He claims it worked. His proof is that he is not only healthier, but far happier.

Is his advice, then, to turn Type A's into Type B's? Friedman asserts that he is not trying to change personalities, but to eliminate what he sees as the destructive side of being a Type A—struggle against time and other people, which creates the hormonal disturbances that lead to disease. "A person can be a Type A but not struggle," he says. "A tiger asleep is the same as a lamb asleep. It's when he awakens that the trouble begins."

Here is what Friedman and Rosenman prescribe:

EVALUATE YOUR STRENGTHS AND WEAKNESSES CANDIDLY
Ask yourself whether your real interests are being satisfied, whether your abilities are being realized. Be realistic about your ambitions.

RETRIEVE YOUR TOTAL PERSONALITY Are you so caught up in acquiring more and more that you leave no room for intellectual or spiritual pursuits? Set aside a portion of each day for pleasures entirely unrelated to your vocation.

ESTABLISH LIFE GOALS Ask yourself exactly what you wish to accomplish in your work and your private life. Commit each set of goals to paper and review them often.

RECOGNIZE THE VALUE OF RITUALS AND TRADITIONS Type A's often consider simple pleasures like holiday dinners a waste of time. Remember you are a social and spiritual being as well as an achiever.

SET PRIORITIES Type A's often devote equal time to the important and the trivial. Insecurity and competitiveness can make them unable to delegate responsibilities; failure is so loathsome they have to keep proving themselves, even with trifles.

REVISE YOUR DAILY SCHEDULE Eliminate as many activities as possible that do not contribute to your socioeconomic well-being. Allot more time for each event than you think it requires; in this way you won't get so cluttered up that you fall victim to hurry sickness. Wake up fifteen minutes earlier so you have time to reflect, take a walk, or eat leisurely; have your secretary keep away unessential phone calls and visitors; don't schedule meetings too close together. Learn to say no.

WORK IN A MILIEU THAT PROMOTES PEACE A's typically have disordered surroundings, which enhances the sense of time urgency. Keep your environment orderly and aesthetically pleasing; objects of beauty and elegance help settle the mind.

CONSIDER YOUR WORDS Most A's talk too much, too narrowly about their own interests. Let others have their say, *and listen.*

BREAK IT AT LUNCHTIME A's tend to work at lunch, scribbling on napkins or gulping down a sandwich at their desks. Cut down on luncheons in which you talk and think of the same things you have in mind the rest of the day. Allot time for an amble in the park, a museum, or window-shopping.

FORGET THE 5:00 FRENZY The battle against time is often self-imposed; A's like to procrastinate until the very last minute so they can compete against the clock. Organize your day so everything gets done without panic.

SPEND SOME TIME ALONE Scan each week in advance and reserve periods of time to be with yourself. Use the time for reflection, or for things you have been meaning to get around to—reading *War and Peace,* writing letters to old friends, playing the piano, etc.

REENGINEER YOUR HOSTILITY Most often, free-floating hostility is a reflection of the longing for love and affection; it is connected with fear. Avoid people who easily stir your anger. If you must see them, use your sense of humor and your good sense—life is here to enjoy, not to annoy.

Behavior Modification for Type A's

Despite Friedman's disclaimer, some critics feel that he is, indeed, trying to turn A's into B's. One such skeptic is Dr. Howard Glazer, a New York psychologist with a private practice and director of behavior management systems at EHE/StressControl Systems, Inc. Glazer is concerned about the possibilities of mistaking behavior pattern for personality type. "You can't make a Type A into a Type B any more than you can make an alcoholic into a non-alcoholic," says Glazer. "You can make them into reformed alcoholics, reformed Type A's, but in both cases, the impulse to destructive behavior has to be controlled."

Behaviorists favor strengthening the Type A's defenses rather than breaking them down, as most psychoanalysts would do. By actually putting the Type A person *more* in control, a well-structured behavior program could promote change without raising the person's anxiety about losing control.

Glazer performed a pilot study at Montreal General Hospital, using behavioral techniques on a number of Type A's. According to preliminary data, he says, the procedures are "highly effective in bringing about the desired changes in life-style." Essentially, he proposes to get the Type A person to use, or redirect those traits to his advantage.

The program that Glazer employs at StressControl Systems, Inc., works best under the guidance of a qualified behavioral psychologist, but it can be employed on your own with reasonable success—if you stick to it.

Keep a "Daily Strain Budget." For two weeks, monitor each activity from the time of awakening. On a scale from one to ten, rate each task according to (1) how much effort was involved and (2) how much tension you felt while performing it. The effort score for each activity is multiplied by its duration (30 minutes equals one unit), and by the tension score. The resulting figure indicates the degree of strain experienced in a single day.

After you have become proficient at calculating daily strain scores, you must determine your own "strain budget." Set your own limits. Then, by juggling the number of activities, their duration, and the effort exerted, see if you can keep within your budget.

At StressControl, subjects are also taught coping techniques to reduce the tension levels of their activities. These include exercise, relaxation procedures, and assertion training, which is used to help regulate interpersonal pressures.

Set up contingency contracts with yourself to reinforce appropriate behavior. These are tied to your daily strain budget. For example, by reducing your score from 500 to 490, you can reward yourself with an hour's worth of recreation. By setting your own reinforcement standards, you can always remain in control.

how to set priorities

One of the keys to eliminating destructive Type A behavior is to learn to set priorities. Here, in brief, is the procedure advocated by Alan Lakein, the time-management consultant whose book, *How to Get Control of Your Time and Your Life* (Signet paperback), has been a boon for many a time-hassled executive.

At the top of a sheet of paper, write, "What are may lifetime goals?"
Take two minutes to list your answers. They should be general and abstract, taking into account personal, family, career, financial, and other goals. Include everything that comes to mind.
Now take an additional two minutes to make changes.
Write on top of another sheet, "How would I like to spend the next three Years?"
Take two minutes and list all those short-term goals.
Take an additional two minutes to add some more.
Now ask, "If I knew I would be struck dead by lightning six months from now, how would I live until then?"
Take two minutes and write. Don't ponder.
Take another two minutes to revise.
Now take at least two minutes to review and improve all three lists. You may find confirmation of the way you are spending your time, or you may find conflicts.
Now take your lifetime goals and select the top three.
Do the same for the other lists.
Using the nine items as your guide, write on a separate paper, "My three most important long-term goals are ..." and list them.
In a few days, and every so often subsequently, revise the list.
Decide on specific activities for achieving long-term goals. Without regard to practicality, write many possible activities for achieving your three goals. Use a separate sheet for each goal.
Go back over your lists, adding, deleting, refining.
You should have far too many activities and not enough time. Now set your priorities; this is the time to be practical.
For each activity ask yourself, "Am I committed to spending time on this activity in the next seven days?" If no, cross it out.
You should end up with at least four activities you consider meaningful and are ready to spend time on next week.
Combine the results into one list; order your priorities.
Classify the most important as A-1. This is the best use of your time. Label the next most important A-2, and so on.
They should be short and feasible; if they are not, divide them into segments.
Set a deadline for each and schedule them for next week.
Get to one of them right away.

self-help procedures

For the most part, mental and emotional difficulties encountered by executives can be handled without professional intervention, if you are willing to own up to your situation honestly, and to make an effort to change. Certain recurrent emotions are precursors of serious disorders and can be nipped in the bud.

Feelings such as anxiety and depression, unless severe and chronic, should not require psychiatric aid. The understanding and support of a close friend, one's spouse, or a circle of colleagues is often sufficient. But many executives live in a vacuum; the higher their position, the more isolated they are. Consequently, virtually every expert has advised executives to cultivate relationships—even just one—in which they can be perfectly candid without fear of reprisal or stigma.

Minor anxiety or depression are signals. Don't treat them as problems in themselves; they are merely signs of hidden conflicts or unresolved emotions that can spiral into more serious mental or physical disorders unless dealt with effectively. Honest introspection, perhaps with a friend or counselor, will help you recognize the roots of the difficulty.

The underlying needs or frustrations upon which negative moods are built should be dealt with when they first arise. If you let them accumulate, your energy will be sapped, the negativity will build, and you can quickly lose both your perspective and your ability to deal with the situation. In addition, pent-up emotions are likely to erupt inappropriately. Don't try to sustain self-confrontation indefinitely.

Emotional problems can be triggered by a variety of factors, but three common overlapping categories should be well understood: self-doubt, fear, and loss.

Self-doubt

Christopher Hegerty, one of the country's leading business consultants, holds that many executives lack self-esteem deep within, despite their professional competence. This, he believes, is largely due to equating our value as human beings with outer achievements. He suggests asking yourself the following questions, honestly, to get an idea of your own self-esteem.

---

self-evaluation: hegerty self-esteem scale

	Yes	No
I often feel inadequate to handle new situations.		
I habitually condemn myself for my mistakes and shortcomings.		
I have a driving need to prove my worth and excellence.		
I am much concerned with what others think and say of me.		
I am prone to condemn others and often wish them punished.		

Yes   No

*I tend to belittle my own talents, possessions, and
    achievements.*
*I feel quite vulnerable to others' opinions, comments,
    and attitudes.*
I am a professional people pleaser.
I have a deep need to gossip about others.
*I often blame others for my handicaps, problems, and
    mistakes.*
I am a compulsive perfectionist.
*I customarily judge my self-worth by personal
    comparison with others.*

If you answered "yes" to a significant number of statements, says
Hegerty, you probably have a serious deficiency in self-esteem.

Experts feel that unconscious self-doubt is the cause of many interpersonal difficulties at work and home, erupting in aggressiveness,
selfishness, hostility, competitiveness, and other abrasive traits that
can trigger the stress response in oneself and others. It can seriously
damage performance as well. Says Dr. Harry Levinson, "Self-doubt is
probably the greatest crippler of executive ability."

It manifests, says the psychologist, in two conspicuous ways:

*Inability to trust yourself to undertake responsibilities for which you
    are qualified and capable. Even a position or assignment to which
    you aspire can be avoided because of underlying fear of failure.*
*The feeling that you have reached an occupational dead-end. This is
    common in the so-called mid-life crisis, discussed later in this
    chapter.*

Levinson recommends the following steps to erase self-doubt (we
paraphrase):
1. Recognize that self-doubt is widespread. You are not alone.
2. Recognize that there is no alternative to perseverance except failure. Whether it means changing jobs or forging ahead in your
   present occupation you must persevere if you are ever to prove
   yourself to your own satisfaction. If you need inspiration pick up
   a biography of any great person. (See following box.)
3. When you find yourself unduly aloof, hostile, compliant, or competitive, you may be acting on the basis of self-doubt. Realize this
   and find more constructive ways to deal with it.
4. If, despite your efforts, your self-doubt keeps you down, makes
   you too defensive, or results in psychosomatic symptoms, it
   might well be time to see a psychiatrist or psychologist.

Psychiatrist Sidney Lecker observes that self-doubt results from failure to live up to one's own standards, which are often unrealistic or imposed from outside. Doubt can lead either to giving up or to impulsive overreaction. Guilt fuels the former, inadequacy feeds the latter.

Lecker suggests standing aside and assessing your feelings objectively. Is your guilt based on any actual infraction? By what standards (or whose) do you come up inadequate? If you can answer those questions and judge yourself favorably, you should be able to absolve yourself of a lot of self-doubt, most of which is irrational.

---

a case history to alleviate self-doubt

If you ever doubt that perseverence can overcome obstacles, or that greatness is often preceded by adversity, consider this biographical sketch of a politician:

1832-lost job
1832-defeated for legislature
1833-failed in private business
1834-elected to legislature
1835-sweetheart dies
1836-nervous breakdown
1836-defeated for house speaker
1843-defeated for nomination to Congress
1846-elected to Congress
1848-lost renomination
1849-ran for land officer and lost
1854-defeated for Senate
1856-defeated for nomination for Vice-President
1858-defeated for Senate again
1860-elected President of the United States.

The politician was, of course, Abraham Lincoln.

Fear

If we could peer inside the mind of a heart-attack or ulcer victim, we would probably find a beehive of worry, most of which is based on exaggerated, unnecessary, or irrational fear. Robert T. Archibald, first vice-president of a large West Coast brokerage firm, learned a lot from his heart attack and subsequent surgery: "I suggest to any executive," he now says, "that 60 to 70 percent of the things we worry about are really insignificant. I now refuse to run for an airplane on a business trip, and I no longer race to see how many branch offices I can visit in a day."

Upon serious inspection, most executives would probably agree—we tend to waste too much time and energy worrying about things that simply don't warrant it. There is an important distinction between concern and worry. To be concerned is to take interest in something of real importance; to worry is to be troubled by, or to struggle with, a possibility that is threatening, but not yet real. The latter never solved a problem: it cripples judgement, destroys perspective, and hampers performance. And it eats away at the stomach and blood vessels.

If you are a habitual worrier, it might be wise to cultivate what Bertrand Russell called "the habit of thinking of the right things at the right time." Don't get bogged down in idle speculation about things outside your control. Avoid needless worry over events that are inevitable. "The wise man thinks about his troubles only when there is some purpose in doing so," wrote Russell. "At other times he thinks about other things. . . . When misfortune threatens, consider seriously and deliberately what is the very worst that could possibly happen. Having looked this possible misfortune in the face, give yourself sound reasons for thinking that after all it would be no such very terrible disaster."

Perceiving problems not as threats but as opportunities or challenges, fosters creative action and keeps ulcers away. Napoleon Hill, author of the bestselling *Think and Grow Rich,* maintains that the subconscious will "translate into reality a thought driven by fear just as readily as it will translate into reality a thought driven by courage or faith. . . . Kill the habit of worry, in all its forms, by reaching a general, blanket decision that nothing which life has to offer is worth the price of worry. With this decision will come poise, peace of mind, and calmness of thought which will bring happiness."

Loss

A good portion of emotional life centers around loss. Anticipated loss causes anxiety, present loss causes pain, remembered loss causes anger and frustration. All three cause physiological imbalances that can lead to serious illness. Coming to terms with loss in one of its three stages is an important feature of mental health, but it is not always easy.

Psychiatrist David Viscott, author of several popular books, including *Risking,* feels that one must confront loss directly. If you fear a loss is about to happen, figure out what is going to occur and make a plan to alter or cope with it. If you are hurting from a loss, you have to go through the pain without denial, excuses, or pretense and try to keep from losing more than necessary. If you are angry over previous loss, you must confront that anger and accept it.

Viscott warns that the process of coping is not pleasant, and that there are no shortcuts. Defenses create blind spots that make it difficult to understand the nature of the loss. But the most damaging thing you can do, he contends, is to hold back unpleasant feelings from expression. When you do that you divide yourself in half—a part that feels and a part that is afraid to feel.

A little honest introspection will help you determine what your own tendencies are. Learning to deal appropriately with loss—real or imagined, past, present, or future—is an important step toward preventing stress disorders.

Viscott notes three kinds of defenses, corresponding to specific character types. The *dependent* person uses denial as a defense. He is, in effect, saying "go away" to his problems. He tends to be concerned with the loss of love; he fears being abandoned.

The *controlling* person's defense is making excuses. He blames other people or circumstances for his problems. He constantly thinks, "If only ..." He is usually concerned with loss of control.

The *competitive* person's defense is pretending. He pretends that things are the way he wishes they were. He does not—like the person who denies—keep all the pain out of his awareness, but he is likely to turn away from it. He is usually concerned with a loss of esteem. He fears being embarrassed by having his shortcomings and pretenses exposed.

---

the mid-life crisis

Sometime between ages 39 and 42, most people leap from early adulthood into middle age. It can be a delicate time, usually accompanied by a concrete emotional reaction, that, left unattended, can lead to physiological problems. For some it may only engender mild introspection, perhaps some self-doubt. For others, it can be a time of intense depression, even accompanied by thoughts of suicide. It is a time when most executives reach a career plateau. It can seem that there is nowhere to go, either financially or in terms of responsibility and challenge.

Says sociologist Charlotte Darrow, quoted in the Summer 1977 issue of *Directors & Boards;* "By age forty, a man has reached his horizon. Whatever illusions he may have held before, this is inevitably a time of assessment. He knows fairly clearly where he has placed in life's battles—and just about how much further he can go."

In *Passages,* the bestselling book based on the theories of psychologist Daniel J. Levinson, author Gail Sheehy analyzed adult life stages. The mid-life period, she says, is one of those potentially traumatic transitions where creative introspection—not typically an executive strong point—is necessary, and new coping devices are called for. Until then, one tends to glide on the hopes and ideals of youth. Now, time and choices are narrowing. Alternatives fade, and so do dreams, as one realizes he or she may never do the things once planned.

At this time, failures may stand out in stark relief. Self-image may suffer as a result. "I am not the person I always wanted to be," thinks the mid-lifer. The result is often deep depression, and the usual antidote —hope—is difficult to swallow since time and youth appear to be on the wane. Anxiety may also result, if the person struggles to avoid an inner confrontation.

The pervasiveness of mid-life crisis is another good reason for having a company psychologist. At such a time, an executive may seriously need someone to talk to, someone who can recognize what is going on and bring it to his attention. Sometimes, a good honest chat is enough to assuage the crisis. Knowing that what you are going through is common, predictable, and understood, can make all the difference.

Reportedly, the mid-life crisis has a happy ending for the executive who can accept himself and his limitations: self-assurance, purpose, and a sense of peace are the result. Experts advise the 40-year-old to edge away from competitiveness and become more of a mentor. Although for some people, and for some organizations, this is a difficult transition, it will benefit both.

---

how to survive mid-life change

StressControl's Sidney Lecker suggests the following steps for handling what he prefers to call mid-life "awakening":

1. Reduce the number of changes you attempt at any one time.
2. Reduce the time pressure—take more, not fewer, rest stops, despite your fear that time is running out.
3. Increase your ability to cope by focusing on the key needs revealed by your mid-life awakening. If for example, your marriage is in need of renewal, attend to that, not more superfluous needs.
4. Rehearse the solution to your needs. Don't act impulsively; discuss and contemplate.
5. Implement your top priorities without fear or guilt.
6. Unload unnecessary stress by relaxing and demobilizing effort that is not needed. Don't make things worse by overdoing it.

The Natural Way to Stress Control, Sidney Lecker (New York: Grosset & Dunlap, 1978).

interpersonal relations

Difficult relations with one's boss, colleagues, and subordinates can be a major source of stress overload. Negative interaction frequently triggers the stress response in situations that, of course, call for neither fight nor flight.

Anger is especially lethal. Most of us do not know how to express anger effectively, thus creating further tension within ourselves and in others. In many cases, we hold it in, perhaps not consciously recognizing the emotion at all. This will keep the stress hormones active, silently wearing down organs and blood vessels.

A typical response for an angry individual is to suppress the feeling and withdraw from whoever set it off. Then, feeling guilty about being angry over some mistake or decision, he will avoid the person, pretend to be jovial, and hope it will go away. But it doesn't, and he ends up quibbling over minor matters, taking it out on his secretary or his family, or developing psychosomatic problems: chronic tension, headaches, ulcers, or worse. Eventually, the pent-up anger can explode in a fit of violence over some relative trifle, thus further contaminating the atmosphere.

For these reasons, experts advise becoming aware of the common sources of anger in your life. Perhaps it is tardiness, insubordination, carelessness, or any of a variety of common irritants, some trivial and some important. Learn you particular bugaboos. Recognize also the early warning signs of anger. Some people get tense in the base of the neck, others lose their appetites, still others develop tightness in the arm and leg muscles.

When you spot the signs of anger, be sure to identify exactly what you are angry about. Was it the fact that the report was late, or that he didn't seem to care about inconveniencing you? If you decide that your anger is justified, rehearse in advance how to handle it. Wait until you cool off; don't let emotions impair your judgement. If confrontation is necessary try to understand the other person's perspective, and then tell him exactly how you feel—calmly, sincerely, and with no ambiguity.

Sometimes, confrontation is inappropriate. Here is where other outlets for the flood of fight-or-flight hormones becomes necessary. Vigorous exercise, or even such private forms of release as screaming (where no one can hear you) or beating up your pillow can alleviate some of the discomfort and help prevent antisocial outbursts.

Dealing effectively with *other* people's anger can also save wear and tear on everyone's system. If you are in the wrong, don't be too proud to apologize. Experts explain that both overdoing an apology or lashing back will provoke further attack from an angry individual. You should understand that the expressed reasons for the person's anger are often not the real ones, nor may you be the actual object that provoked the emotion. But, while compassion is vital, so is firmness. Make it clear that you will hear him out, but you won't be a whipping boy.

Assertiveness vs. Aggression

Recognizing the difference between assertiveness and aggression, or hostility, psychologists have devised methods for training people to assert their own feelings and needs while at the same time turning "adversary relationships" into "caring relationships." The following points are taken from the assertion-training portion of a stress-management program at Kaiser-Permanente's Southern California health facility. The material was provided by Don Isbell and Sally Nelson, who developed the program. Follow these points when a potentially stressful situation arises between you and another person. It will help keep the atmosphere harmonious and constructive.

---

communicating

Compose yourself by taking a deep, abdominal breath as described in Chapter eight.

Make eye contact with the person.

Don't go on until you feel relaxed and are sure you will not erupt in rage. If you need more time, use what they call a "zero-scale" response, such as "okay," or "all right."

If you are still unable to relax, it might be best to temporarily remove yourself from the situation. Disengage with a polite statement, such as "I'm really upset now. I'd like to return in a few minutes and talk with you about what happened."

Use "I" statements to express your feelings or make a request. This is to simply let the other person know where you stand, not to give you power leverage.

Reflect the other person's response by using "and" statements, not "but." For example, "I understand you are upset, and when you yell like that, I get very upset." This kind of response, as opposed to the more negative statement using "but," creates an air of conciliation and allows for constructive discussion.

Assess your effect. Did the person hear you? If so, continue. If he or she was too angry to understand, restate or reflect in another way. If it seems that communication is impossible, disengage until another time.

State your needs and your common goals with the person. This can be difficult when anger and defensiveness rule, but it is vital for creating an empathic mood. Example: "I would like to see our

> *department as productive as possible and I know you would like us to try your plan. Here is a suggestion I would like to share with you."*

Assertiveness can be a useful tool for preventing trouble and working out solutions. But it can be abused. Don't turn it into advice giving, one-upsmanship, commiseration, or condescension. Its purpose is not control or oppression, but mutually beneficial collaboration.

In a complex, changing organization, a certain amount of ambiguity is, perhaps, inevitable. Here are some of the ways that authorities like Dr. Levinson recommend for minimizing the anxiety caused by ambiguity and related factors:

Try to plan change together with people who are going to be involved in it.

Maintain continuing contact with subordinates, supporting their efforts, and defining the limits of their task.

Provide the opportunity to talk things over. Give people the opportunity to discuss matters before acting.

Help people realize that feelings like hostility, disappointment, and uncertainty are common in some circumstances.

———— professional help and consultation ————

The old image of the shrink as a grim man with a Mephistophelean beard and a Viennese accent, who plumbs the psychic deeps while his patient lies on a leather couch free-associating, is completely out of date. In-depth analysis is increasingly being limited to persons whose lives are impossibly out of control. For most mild or temporary setbacks, newer forms of therapy—less analytic, less intense, and aimed at definite, short-range objectives—have won the favor of the psychiatric community.

Most psychologists feel that stress-related executive problems seldom require psychoanalysis. For them, behavioral approaches, nonintensive group procedures, transactional analysis, or the "growth therapies" developed by the school of humanistic psychology are probably the better choices.

Choosing a therapist or counselor is no simple matter. Care should be taken and discrimination employed. There are as many bad shrinks as there are bad businessmen. And since psychological counselors and therapists are usually not required to be licensed, there is nothing to prevent virtually anyone from hanging up a shingle.

While it is not essential, or even always desirable, to use a psychiatrist (a therapist with an M.D.), it is wise to select a therapist with a doctorate from a reputable institution. In some cases, individuals with master's degrees in psychology or social work can provide excellent counseling. The qualities that make a good therapist—sincerity, empathy, and the ability to communicate and provide insight—can really not be taught in school.

The best way to select a therapist is to obtain a reference from a reliable and trusted source. Your physician should be able to recommend one, as will your local medical society or mental health association. The American Psychiatric Association has state branches that keep records of qualified therapists. Other sources include your local hospital's psychiatric department, medical schools, or the psychology department of a university.

In addition, there are several reference sources. *The Directory of Approved Counseling Agencies* provides a complete list of accredited agencies from which you can obtain quality therapy. *A Complete Guide To Therapy: From Psychoanalysis to Behavior Modification,* by Dr. Joel Kovel, summarizes all the options available and describes the various forms of therapy. For "growth centers" and more unusual forms of therapy, write to the Association for Humanistic Psychology, 325 Ninth St., San Francisco, Calif. 94103.

mental health services for corporations

Psychiatrists have long been associated with corporations. But until recently, their main purpose was to screen out unstable employees, weed out problem drinkers, and occasionally add their two cents on promotion decisions. More recently, their roles have expanded.

Just how much should a company meddle in its employees' mental and emotional lives? Some feel that it is intrusive and a breach of privacy to become involved. Others feel that "the job" is often a major source of difficulty, and the office is a perfect place to identify problems before they get out of hand. This school believes that mental health should be on an equal footing with medical care. This latter school is winning out, as an increasing number of experts are being called in to provide not just counseling and treatment, but prevention. Their job in many instances is to promote mental health, harmony, and happiness within a relatively stress-free environment.

In some cases, a large company will hire a staff psychiatrist or psychologist, on either a full or part-time basis. Sometimes the company nurse will be given special training in dealing with simple emotional problems. Employee assistance programs, growing in popularity among government agencies, provide short-term counseling on issues such as divorce, marital difficulties, and problems with supervisors or co-workers. The fastest growing trend, however, is the use of outside consultants. The services provided by these organizations range from stress-prevention programs to long-term counseling for disturbed individuals. The following pages outline the services offered by five of the larger and more popular organizations servicing the corporate world: Forbes Associates, The Levinson Institute, The Center for Applied Behavioral Sciences, EHE StressControl Systems, and Life Extension Institute Psychological Services.

**Forbes Associates
9 South Downing Street
Denver, Colo. 80200**

Over the past eight years, Dr. Rosalind Forbes has worked with executives from sixty corporations to help them channel stress into a "positive management force." Her clients include Xerox, United Airlines, Chase Manhattan Bank, AT&T, and the American Management Association, whom she serves out of her offices in Denver. Dr. Forbes and her associates provide individually designed stress-management programs to corporations. They are not clinical psychologists, and do not provide therapy. Theirs is an educationally oriented program emphasizing prevention. "We're not out to remove stress," says Dr. Forbes, "but to change people's reactions to it, so that the locus of control is within themselves."

---

forbes associates services

Forbes Associates' programs include the following basic features:

A preliminary work-up of the organization and each participant, using survey methods to identify environmental stress factors.
Physiological stress profiles of each participant to ascertain tension levels and visceral responses to stress.
15–40 hours of training in half-day sessions tailored to the company's work schedule. These include relaxation procedures, biofeedback, breathing, and stretching exercises.
Seminars on principles of stress management.
Consultation and record keeping to help recognize individual stress responses and patterns.
Group sessions for sharing of common problems and individual counseling for persons with special psychological or medical problems.
Individual tapes and charts for use at home and work.
Use of biofeedback machines twice weekly following the workshops.

Follow-up sessions including surveys and physiological profiles designed to measure progress.

The Levinson Institute, Inc.
Box 95
Cambridge, Mass. 02138

Founded by Dr. Harry Levinson after fourteen years as director of the Division of Industrial Mental Health at the Menninger Foundation, the Levinson Institute is one of the giants in corporate mental health. It is an association of psychologists and psychiatrists "dedicated to helping organizations and the people in them adapt effectively to competitive and changing environments."

Week-long seminars are conducted in the Boston area, which bring together executives from diverse organizations. The same seminars can also be provided for from twenty to forty executives in an organization's own setting. Both types have been attended by top executives of major corporations. The in-house seminars range from 2 1/2 to 5 days, and the cost varies with duration and distance from Boston. The cost of one weekly seminar, including instruction, books, meals, and lodging at the Sheraton Rolling Green Inn, 40 minutes from Boston, is $1450.

levinson seminars

The Levinson Institute Seminars are designed to help executives–

Understand and discharge their leadership roles effectively
Anticipate and manage change in ways that are healthy and adaptive
Exercise authority with less frustration and anguish
Make psychologically sound decisions
Assess psychological consequences of managerial decisions
Use themselves effectively in the development of subordinates and the management of groups
Understand what contributes to executive stress and alleviate those pressures
Understand the predictable stages of executive career development and planning

The seminars conducted include:
1. *On Leadership*
2. *The Modern Organization*
3. *Managing Stress and Change in Organizations*
4. *Coaching, Counseling, and Consultation*

5. *The Executive Couple*
The Levinson Institute also offers consultation services, emphasizing the diagnosis of problems. These consultation services include:
1. *Top Management Counsel*
2. *Executive Crisis Counseling*
3. *Conflict Resolution*
4. *Executive Selection*
5. *Organizational Design*
6. *Termination Processes*
7. *Retirement and Transitional Counseling*
8. *Organizational Diagnosis*
9. *Organizational Processes*
10. *Organizational Development*

The Levinson Institute also publishes books on the seminar subjects, conducts research studies, and distributes the *Levinson Letter,* a biweekly newsletter on the psychological aspects of organizational life.

Center for Applied Behavioral Sciences
The Menninger Foundation
Box 829
Topeka, Kansas 66601

The Menninger Foundation is a renowned center for psychiatric treatment, education, research, and social application. The Center For Applied Behavioral Sciences (CABS) was begun in 1956 by the late Dr. William C. Menninger as the Division of Industrial Mental Health. Since then, more than 2000 companies and 20,000 participants have taken advantage of their seminars, workshops, consultation services, and special projects.

The center's principal seminar is entitled "Toward Understanding Human Behavior and Motivation." Intended to provide insight that will "enhance satisfaction and fulfillment in work and family lives," it incorporates lectures, structured groups, and individual meetings. Four dimensions of behavior are addressed:

How the individual experiences himself and the world
Principles of interaction with other persons
How individuals function in groups, and how groups operate
How subgroups within an organization interact

Reporter Lawrence Maloney of *U.S. News and World Report,* attended one of the seminars. He writes: "There is no pressure on anyone to reveal more than he or she wants to. Still, the businessmen do let down their hair in a way many never do in their everyday lives. Discussions turn up worries over marital problems, coping with children, frustrations on the job, and friction between executives and their employees...."

The prinicipal seminar is offered in three different five-day formats: Executive Seminar ($1500); Young Executive Seminar ($1000); and Government Executive Seminar ($800). They include individual interviews and psychological assessment. In addition, there is a condensed three-day Executive Seminar for those whose schedules do not permit a five-day stay. It costs $750 and additional discounts are provided for companies that send three or more executives.

For those who have attended the basic seminar, an Advanced Executive Seminar is offered ($1000). Stress-reduction exercises are practiced, the emotions displayed in everyday business are addressed, videotape feedback is used, and each participant works on a thorough life-assessment with the professional staff.

Alumni of the basic seminar may also attend the Advanced Seminar for Executive Couples, which costs no more per couple than the per-person cost. Its goal is creating balance between work and family, covering such areas as the feelings of a spouse of an executive devoted to the company, the guilt of the executive whose schedule disallows time for the family, and relocation or job transition.

The Executive Seminar may also be taken on a seven-day whitewater wilderness rafting trip. Conducted by a team from the foundation along with an experienced Outward Bound staff, the expedition is conducted in Colorado and Utah. Tuition for this exhilarating journey is $1600, including all food, supplies, camping equipment, and local transportation.

The center also provides contracted seminars, held either in Topeka or on the client company's own site. Enrollment is limited to those designated by the client, who may choose specific seminar themes. Members of the center staff are also available to speak at annual meetings, conferences, and conventions.

center consulting services

The Center for Applied Behavioral Sciences also offers a wide range of consulting services:

Executive Consultations Life assessment, career development, retirement planning, promotions, work-family interplay, and other potentially troublesome areas are covered. Some companies offer this service to executives every three to five years as a voluntary part of their annual health examination. They usually last one to two days and utilize an interdisciplinary team of consultants. Spouses are encouraged to participate.

> *Organizational Consultation* This includes informal counseling, staff training, organizational development, and referral services to assist companies in three major areas: diagnosing potential conflicts caused by management systems and employees under stress, staff training programs, and intervention where serious conflicts have developed.

EHE StressControl Systems, Inc.
210 E. 49th St.
New York, N.Y. 10017

This relatively new wing of Executive Health Examiners is a pioneer in the field, an attempt to link stress programs run by mental health experts with regular medical services. Its director is psychiatrist Sidney Lecker, who is accompanied by a staff of psychologists in different areas of specialization.

---

ehe stresscontrol systems

CrisisSupport System Available only to registered clients, this service attempts to minimize the effects of crisis on the victim and co-workers. Clients can use a "hot line" to the StressControl Center for information to reduce risk and discomfort, for arranging emergency care, for priority appointments with Center psychologists, and for advice on coping with the crisis. ($150 registration, $100/hour for service.)

StressCope System One-to-one counseling is provided for employees whose performance has declined and whose employment is in jeopardy. The supervisor will be advised on what to say to the person and how to arrange for consultation. ($450 for evaluation plus three hours counseling and reports; follow-up is $300.)

StressManagement System This service will identify the amount and sources of stress on the employee and improve his ability to cope with it. The focus is the StressManagement Examination personality questionnaires highlighting areas of stress and its intensity, and biofeedback monitoring of physiologic responses to stress. ($75/hour.) EHE hopes to make the StressManagement Examination a regular part of its physical examinations.

StressPrevention System An educational service to help employees through job-induced or personal transitions. Individual training is provided in relaxation methods. Group seminars discuss stress and its effects according to each organization's needs and interests.

StressControl's most widely used service is consultation with individuals about to undergo the trauma of relocation. Experts evaluate the ability of the candidate and his family to handle the move, and counsel them on how to minimize the impact.

If your organization already has a medical unit, and you wish to provide rudimentary psychological services, StressControl will provide stress management training to nurses and counselors. The center also has a Division on Women and Stress, headed by Dr. Carol Beauvais, a clinical psychologist. In addition to its New York facility, StressControl Systems maintains a national network of associated consultants that is particularly useful to clients with multiple locations.

Life Extension Institute Psychological Services
1185 Avenue of the Americas
New York, N.Y. 10020

This is a relatively new addition to the LEI medical program. It consists of private consultation with the LEI professional staff for evaluation and referral for treatment as required. Follow-up is included.

Any individual with an emotional or medical-behavioral problem, or anyone who would like to reduce some negative emotional response such as anger or hostility, may utilize the services of LEI psychiatrists, psychologists, physicians, educators, and counselors. The basic charge is $75 for one hour or any part thereof, and $50 for any part of a subsequent hour. Individualized programs may include behavior modification, biofeedback, hypnosis, systematic desensitization, and relaxation therapies.

LEI's *Employees Assistance Program* provides means of identification, referral, treatment, and follow-up for troubled employees (such as alcoholics) whose work performance has deteriorated seriously. The program includes written statements of policies and procedures, endorsement by top-level management, management involvement, uniform identification and referral policy, company-wide educational and informational service, and training supervisors to understand treatment and follow-up procedures.

Dr. Charles M. Rose of InterHealth, the San Diego affiliate of LEI, in collaboration with the U.S. Naval Health Research Center, has designed a computerized Stress Profile that will soon be added to LEI's services. For $10—added to the cost of a regular physical, or taken as a separate service—the individual will fill out an extensive questionnaire, which will be fed into a computer for quantitative evaluation of several psychological variables. The score on each scale will be compared with norms for the average population, and a risk factor will be computed for various aspects of mental health. The subsequent report will indicate methods for improving areas that seem to require attention. When the service is instituted, consultation—either group or individual—will be provided so that the reports can be properly understood and interpreted.

—————— recommended reading: chapter 5 ——————

Depression: A Layman's Guide to the Symptoms and Cures, Paul Gillette (New York: Dutton, 1973).

Executive Stress, Harry Levinson (New York: Harper & Row, 1970).

How To Lick Executive Stress, Robert Collier Page (New York: Cornerstone Library, 1977).

Our Inner Conflicts, Karen Horney (New York: Norton, 1945).

Passages, Gail Sheehy (New York: Dutton, 1976).

Psychosomatic Diagnosis, Flanders Dunbar (New York: Harper, 1943).

Risking, David Viscott (New York: Simon & Schuster, 1978).

Self-Rescue, John Kantwell Kiley (New York: McGraw-Hill, 1977).

The Conquest of Happiness, Bertrand Russell (New York: Liveright, 1930).

The Meaning of Anxiety, Rollo May (New York: Ronald Press, 1950).

The Natural Way to Stress Control, Sidney Lecker (New York: Grosset & Dunlap, 1978).

The Public Affairs Committee publishes a number of fine pamphlets on stress and mental health related areas. Write for a brochure: Public Affairs Committee, 38 Park Avenue, New York, N.Y. 10016.

Think and Grow Rich, Napoleon Hill (Greenwich, Conn.: Fawcett, 1960).

Type A Behavior and Your Heart, Meyer Friedman and Ray Rosenman (New York: Knopf, 1974).

plans, programs and practices

exercise and your health

Exercise is bunk. If you are healthy, you don't need it: if you are sick, you shouldn't take it.—Henry Ford

---

self-evaluation: how do you exercise?

1. Do you exercise regularly? How often?
2. What type of exercise do you do?
3. Do you think of exercise as drudgery, or do you enjoy it?
4. Do you have difficulty fitting exercise into your schedule?
5. Have you been promising yourself that you will get back into shape, but avoiding it?
6. Have you been told by doctors to exercise regularly?
7. Have you been told not to exercise?
8. Do you have any medical condition that limits your participation in vigorous recreation?
9. Do you engage in competitive sports?
10. Do you feel you are too old or out of shape for exercise?
11. Do you ever walk up stairs instead of taking the elevator, just for the exercise?
12. Do you walk instead of taking cabs?
13. Do you ever take walks after work, just for the enjoyment of it?
14. While sitting at your desk, do you ever feel the urge to get up and run around?
15. Do you do mild, stretching exercises, like yoga?

Today, the company gym is almost as common in American business as Ford's assembly line. More than 1000 large corporations have in-house fitness facilities, says the American Foundation of Fitness

Directors for Business and Industry. The elaborate exercise club at Weyerhauser's headquarters in Tacoma, Washington, cost the company $73,000. However, according to *Fortune* magazine, "A modest gym can be set up for about $2000 excluding the costs of space and instructors; the sum would be enough to provide a variety of exercise machines, including an Exercycle and a treadmill for jogging in place."

Companies who have taken the initiative feel the investment was a wise one. They cite greater productivity, better morale, fewer turnovers, and lower sickness and absentee rates. Mostly, however, the push toward exercise—both in and out of the corporate world—is based on the widespread belief that exercise is vital for staving off disease, especially heart disease. The sedentary businessman, with the fight-or-flight response triggered many times a day, is said to need the exercise more than most.

Thus, at General Foods' headquarters outside New York City, all 40 top executives engage in weekly workouts. Supervised by company medical personnel, Exxon's executives spend an hour three times a week going through a series of ten exercise stations. According to a *Newsweek* report, employees of *Forbes* magazine are urged to use the company gym, and those who don't are often reprimanded by their colleagues. At most companies, facilities are simply made available and executives are encouraged to use them.

why exercise?

Mental and spiritual fitness, both dependent on a good brain, are greatly enhanced by optimal physical fitness. Body, mind, and soul are inextricably woven together, and whatever helps or hurts any one of these three sides of the whole man helps or hurts the other two.
—Cardiologist Paul Dudley White

We have more than 600 muscles in our body. They were meant to be used; they thrive on movement, and in its absence they deteriorate. And since our muscles not only enable us to walk, run, lift, and carry, but also to push food through the digestive track, suck air into the lungs, contract or dilate blood vessels, and pump blood through the body, if they are not working efficiently, any and all bodily functions can be adversely affected.

One former president of the American Medical Association said, "It begins to appear that exercise is the master conditioner for the healthy and the major therapy for the ill." He is not alone in his conviction. Dr. Jesse L. Steinfel, former U.S. Surgeon General, says of exercise, "It will make you more effective in your work and at the same time bring personal compensations, one of which is that exercise appears to retard the aging process."

Here are some of the specific benefits noted by physicians:

increased strength and endurance (leads to more efficient use of energy
even in mental tasks)
maintains proper circulation
increased poise and grace
improved muscle tone and posture
reduction of chronic tiredness
reduction of chronic tension
improved control of weight
reduced aches, pains, stiffness
fewer serious accidents
improved appearance
reduction of degenerative disease risk factors

Some benefits, of course, are multilayered. If exercise helps control weight, for example, it will have a direct effect on diseases to which the obese are especially vulnerable, such as diabetes, arthritis, and heart disease. According to studies by the Harvard School of Public Health, half an hour of proper exercise each day can keep off or take off as much as 26 pounds a year.

Even simple, everyday forms of exercise can help. Says Dr. Stare: "The sedentary businessman especially should make exercise a part of his daily life. He ought to get into the habit, for instance, of walking instead of taking cabs for short rides. He ought to walk up a flight or two of stairs at the office, instead of always taking the elevator."

Such a plan has worked, for instance, for Eugene J. Sullivan, president of Borden, Inc. He says he lost ten pounds in a year simply by briskly walking twenty blocks to his office each day. John Connor, chairman of Allied Chemical Corp., stays at a trim 175 pounds with fifteen minutes of in-place jogging and exercises morning and night. "I also avoid sweets," he adds, a reminder that a combination of exercise and diet is crucial for weight loss.

Few, if any, significant benefits can be gained from such simple exercises as a few minutes of push-ups and sit-ups in the morning, or walking your dog at night. The important health inplications of exercise on the cardiovascular system that have attracted the greatest attention derive from much more sustained and dynamic activity. It is now widely believed that *aerobics*—jogging, brisk walking, cycling, swimming, and other exercises that raise heart and breath rates—*can* play a major role in preventing heart disease, rehabilitating its victims, and making the impact of heart attacks less severe for those who can't avoid them.

Does Exercise Prevent Heart Disease?

Studies comparing sedentary workers with those whose work is physically strenuous have usually shown that the active workers have fewer heart attacks. However, many other variables are thought to be at work. Further complicating matters is another chicken/egg question: are people healthier because they exercise, or do they exercise because they are healthier?

Dr. Steven M. Horvath, director of the Institute of Environmental Stress in Santa Barbara, California, sums up the prevailing scientific viewpoint:

> It would appear that the burden of proof still rests on those who state physical activity has a protective or even preventive influence on cardiac disease (including hypertension). The inconclusive data suggest some possible long-term cardiovascular benefits resulting from increased physical activity. How much benefit accrues, how effectively the benefit is retained, and how much physical activity is needed to reduce and to prevent cardiovascular disease are open questions.

A recently concluded study may help resolve those questions. Dr. Ralph S. Paffenberger, Jr., an epidemiologist at the Stanford University School of Medicine, studied the histories of some 17,000 subjects. He concluded that men who regularly engaged in strenuous activities—jogging, swimming, tennis—had fewer heart attacks than those who were less active. Those who expended fewer than 2000 calories per week in physical activity had a 64 percent higher risk of heart attack.

The evidence is more convincing, authorities say, in the area of rehabilitation. At one time exercise was strictly forbidden to heart patients. Now it is virtually standard. Dr. Terrance Kavanaugh, medical director of the Toronto Cardiac Rehabilitation Center, who uses exercise with patients who have had heart attacks, reports a 1.4 percent per annum mortality rate. "In groups that don't exercise," says Kavanaugh, "the comparable rate is 6 to 12 percent. And we got those results with 780 patients—probably the biggest exercise coronary rehab group in the world."

If Paffenberger's results are valid it would appear that very *light* exercise, while beneficial in other ways, may be insignificant with respect to heart disease. Reduced risk was found only in those who *regularly* engaged in *strenuous* activity. Reports *New York Times* health writer Jane E. Brody, "Those who participated in 'light' sports like bowling, baseball, biking, boating, and golf, which require comparatively little energy output, were no better off than those who were inactive."

The important point is that in order to reduce heart risk significantly, the persons in the study had to expend at least 2000 calories per week. That means reducing your risk of heart attack through exercise alone would require an hour of singles' tennis (420–480) calories, an hour of squash (660), an hour of cycling at 12 mph (480–600), and an hour of running at 6 mph (660) every week, or a comparable regimen.

What Does Exercise Do for the Heart?

Findings indicate that valuable changes in important physiological processes result from vigorous aerobic-type exercise.

---

benefits of regular vigorous exercise

Blood pressure is lowered.
Resting heart rate is lowered, meaning that the heart does not have to work as hard to get blood to the rest of the body.
Cardiac output is increased, meaning that the heart is better able to distribute blood where needed under stress.
Number of red blood cells is increased, meaning that more oxygen can be carried per quart of blood.
Elasticity of arteries is increased.
Triglyceride level is lowered.
Blood cholesterol level is decreased. High density cholesterol, which is more protective of blood vessels than low density cholesterol, is proportionately increased.
Adrenal secretions in response to emotional stress are lowered.
Lactic acid is more efficiently eliminated from the muscles (this has been associated with decreased fatigue and tension).
Fibrin, a protein that aids in the formation of blood clots, is decreased.
Additional routes of blood supply are built up in the heart.

The last point in the box above is based on two related postulations. Taken together, these form the core of the exercise enthusiasts' hopes for heart disease.

The first possibility is that the body actually grows new blood vessels in order to keep the heart thoroughly oxygenated. Thus, exercise is said to help overcome atherosclerosis by setting up detour routes around clogged arteries. Since most people over 30 have some degree of plaque formation, it is felt that regular, vigorous, gradually stepped-up exercise is essential for preventing oxygen starvation in the heart.

The second possibility is that blood vessels may actually grow in size, thus enabling blood to flow more smoothly. This might explain the lowering of blood pressure and the lowered incidence of heart attack: if the arteries are larger, there is less chance that a clot will obstruct blood flow.

Is there evidence to support these notions? Yes, but not all experts are convinced. Autopsies of well-conditioned men have revealed above-averaged-sized coronary arteries, but these could have been the result of heredity, not exercise.

A recent study by Dr. Ronald Sylvester at the University of Southern California divided a group of 110 men with proven heart disease into four groups ranging from those who were inactive to those who worked out rigorously. Angiograms revealed a direct correlation between exercise rate and the number of subjects whose arteries worsened. In addition, and perhaps more important, there was a strong inverse correlation between exercise and the rate of recurrence of heart attacks.

─────────────────── **exercise and heart attacks** ───────────────────

	Rate of Exercise	% Whose Arteries Worsened	% of Recurrence of Heart Attack
Group I	inactive	More than 50%	33%
Group II	low-level	48%	20%
Group III	moderate	37%	20%
Group IV	high-level	20%	none

"The bottom line on all of this," says Dr. Sylvester, "is that if you get into a training program to prevent coronary-artery disease, the level of training you should be working for is a really high level of fitness training."

Other heart specialists are also sold on exercise, particularly jogging. Dr. Thomas J. Bassler, president of the American Medical Joggers Association, who claims dual expertise on the subject ("I've run 66 marathons and done 3000 autopsies"), believes that anyone who jogs an hour a day six days a week will become immune to heart disease. "You get remodeling of the coronary arteries," he is convinced. "They are torn down and built up another way so that they become bigger."

For the most part, the medical establishment agrees that exercise is good for you, but not all of them approve of colleagues who push people to extremes. They warn those who are out of condition to avoid the dangers inherent in overdoing it, and they caution that *any* exercise program must be started up gradually. Drs. Freidman and Rosenman write:

> Severe exercise may very well kill you instantaneously. But persons of all ages, if they do not suffer already from crippling coronary heart disease should indulge in as much moderate physical activity as they possibly can. Certainly, at least one hour a day and preferably more time should be spent in moving your legs and arms.

exercise and aerobics

You are more likely to stick with an exercise that you enjoy, but keep on with a new one for a month or two before deciding for or against it. "There is no best exercise for everyone," says cardiologist and exercise specialist Lenore R. Zohman. However, not all types of exercise are equally useful to the cardiovascular system. For improving the capacity of the heart and circulatory system, an exercise *must be aerobic.*

Aerobic exercises—running, walking, swimming, cycling, and jogging—cause the heart and lungs to work harder than they normally do by engaging the large muscles of the trunk and legs in vigorous contraction and relaxation. They demand lots of oxygen.

Writes Dr. Kenneth Cooper in one of his bestselling books on aerobics:

> The main objective of an aerobic exercise program is to increase the maximum amount of oxygen that the body can process within a given time. This is called your *aerobic capacity.* It is dependent upon an ability to (1) rapidly breathe large amounts of air, (2) forcefully deliver large volumes of blood, and (3) effectively deliver oxygen to all parts of the body. In short, it depends upon efficient lungs, a powerful heart, and a good vascular system.
>
> Cardiovascular conditioning, or "fitness," has to do with endurance, not muscles, and not calories. The amount of energy (calories) you burn up depends on the amount of work your body does. Conditioning depends on both the amount of work and the vigor with which it is done.

Competitive Sports

Although many competitive sports involve periods during which the participant is engaged in aerobic-type activities, e.g. running, these usually come in spurts. Therefore, the sustained, repetitive value of aerobics is not achieved.

merits of exercises for cardiovascular conditioning

Activity	Calories/Minute	Value
Walking 1–2 mph	2–4	Not strenuous enough, unless your capacity is extremely low
Golfing, power cart	2½–4	Too intermittent, not taxing
Cycling at 6 mph	4–5	Adequate if you have low capacity
Walking at 3.0 mph	4–5	Adequate if you have low capacity
Golfing, pulling cart	4–5	Useful if sufficiently taxing
Walking 3–5 mph	5–6	Good
Cycling at 8 mph	5–6	Good
Badminton, volleyball	5–6	Only if continuous play
Golfing, carrying clubs	5–6	Only if sufficiently taxing
Tennis, doubles	5–6	Not beneficial unless continuous
Calisthenics	5–6	OK if continuous and rhythmic
Walking 4–5 mph	6–8	Very good
Cycling 10–11 mph	6–8	Very good
Tennis, singles	7–8	OK if skilled and keep moving for 30 minutes
Water skiing	7–8	Not good; risky for cardiac prone
Jogging 5 mph	8–10	Excellent endurance builder
Cycling 12 mph	8–10	Excellent
Downhill skiing	8–10	Not good for endurance; may not be good for cardiac prone
Paddleball	8–10	Not continuous enough; may be dangerous to cardiacs
Running 5.5 mph	10–11	Excellent
Cycling 13 mph	10–11	Excellent
Squash or handball (practice or warmup)	10–11	Too intermittent
Running 6–8 mph	11 and up	Excellent
Handball or squash (competetive)	11 and up	Too intermittent; dangerous if not in top condition

Physicians are cautious about competitive sports for the cardiac-prone Type A's because they tend to become overly aggressive, competitive, and hostile, since they tend to pursue achievement and victory with a fury. Said one such executive when asked if he was enjoying his tennis match, "I'm not here to have a good time, I'm here to play tennis." These individuals are likely to push themselves beyond the limits of their capacity for the sake of winning. The result: the very heart attack they are trying to avoid. This pattern can also hold during activities like jogging. They may push themselves to set unreasonable goals for distance and speed.

Therefore, if you fit the Type A pattern, approach your exercise—and all your recreational pursuits—*noncompetitively.* Set no goals, except the ones given to you by your physician or those that fit into the safe guidelines provided by exercise specialists. Never make a contest of aerobics. Don't be cavalier about warnings or ignore obvious signs of impending danger, such as chest pains.

Beginning an Aerobic Program

If you've been an armchair athlete for many years, you must ease into exercise gradually. Take a comprehensive physical, especially if you are over 35; approximately 10 percent of ostensibly normal male adults over age 35 have hidden heart disease, as contrasted with one percent of men below age 35, according to the American Heart Association. Most doctors recommend that sedentary people about to embark on an exercise campaign at least have their blood pressure taken and their blood analyzed for cholesterol and triglycerides.

Especially for those over 35, a physical exam should include an exercise stress test, such as that described in an earlier chapter. It is the best way available to determine the system's response to vigorous exercise. Jogging expert Dr. Kenneth Cooper feels that he can predict severe heart problems with 85 percent accuracy with the treadmill test.

"The resting EKG picks up single-vessel coronary disease only about 15 percent of the time," said Cooper. "The more sophisticated Masters two-step test, in which a person is monitored while taking a step up and a step back, will pick up single-vessel coronary disease only 35 percent of the time. But studies of stress EKG tests—ours and others —indicate that this method will pick up single-vessel problems as high as 93 percent of the time."

Most hospitals and well-equipped clinics can administer the stress test. Some places, such as New York's Cardio-Metrics, Inc., will administer the test for about $150, including consultation and exercise prescription. Wherever you get the exam, the consulting physician will be able to tell you how strenuously you may begin without fear of sudden heart problems. Some will give you an individually designed program.

Under no conditions should anyone with known heart problems, or anyone with high risk factors, begin a serious exercise program without a thorough examination.

At the beginning, it is best to work out every other day, or at least three days a week. Joggers should not go at it every day at the outset —the chances of developing foot or leg problems are too great. It takes time for the bones, ligaments, and muscles to get used to supporting the body while bouncing around. Once they become accustomed to it, switching to daily jogging is acceptable. On off-days, be sure to perform some stretching exercises or calisthenics; take a brisk walk or a swim.

The Target Zone

According to most experts, there is a precise amount of exercise that is enough to achieve fitness, but is not overstrenuous to the point of exceeding safe limits. This "target zone" is between 60 and 80 percent of the person's own *maximal aerobic power,* which is the point beyond which the heart cannot deliver any more oxygen to the tissues. Further demands on the body will produce exhaustion.

The target zone is about 70 to 85 percent of the *maximal attainable heart rate.* One of the values of the exercise stress test is that your doctor will determine each of those values for you. He will be able to tell if your aerobic capacity and maximal attainable heart rate are below normal, indicating the need for restricting your exercise program. If you do not have a stress test, you can determine your own target zone by assuming you are average and consulting the chart below.

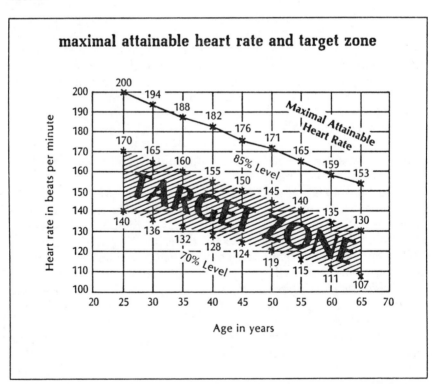

how to measure your heart rate

To determine your heart rate, count your pulse immediately upon stopping exercise. Find the beat quickly, and count it for ten seconds. Then multiply by six to get the count per minute. Because the pulse will fall off sharply once the workout is ended, don't count past the ten seconds.

Whether you jog, run, swim, walk briskly, cycle, run in place, or pedal a stationary bike, you should shoot for about 20 minutes in your target zone. Start with a rate that seems easy for you and do it for 5 to 10 minutes. Stop and take your pulse. It will probably be less than 50 percent of the attainable heart rate for your age group. Then resume the exercise, but more vigorously this time. After 3 to 5 minutes, stop and take your pulse again. If it is below 70 percent of your maximum (the lower limit of your target zone), exercise more strenuously. If it is above 85 percent (the upper limit), exercise less vigorously, either by slowing down or working less hard.

Continue taking your pulse every 5 minutes or so until you have determined what is necessary to put you into the target zone.

The older you get, the lower your maximal aerobic power and maximal attainable heart rate, meaning that an older person can expend the same amount of effort as a younger person without his heartbeat rising quite as high. These numbers on the chart indicate *averages;* Dr. Zohman points out that as many as one-third of the population may deviate from these values.

Dr. Zohman, from whom this procedure was adapted, suggests that you will soon recognize "certain normal sensations you get when you are in the target zone, such as an awareness of a certain amount of rapid heart action or breathlessness." After a while, you should be able to judge what it takes to reach your target zone and when you are in danger of exceeding it, thus eliminating the need for stopping to take your pulse.

Build up gradually. "It takes at least six months for a sedentary man to become a good jogger," warns Dr. Willibald Nagler of Cornell's College of Medicine in New York. "Just don't make any sudden changes in your exercise routine."

As you develop, you will find that the exercise will go more easily. You will have to exert more energy to reach your target zone, because your heart will not have to work as hard to maintain the same level of energy. Thus, reevaluate yourself every few weeks and upgrade your routine accordingly. Keep a running record of your heart rate at rest, after warming up, during and after your workout.

Keep in mind that you have to continue aerobics on a regular basis in order to maintain effectiveness. "If you cut back to exercising once a week, half of your fitness increase will be lost in a mere ten weeks," warns Dr. Zohman. "If you discontinue your program completely, all your gains will be lost in five weeks."

If you are traveling, or if you become ill, or for any other reason are forced to discontinue for a while, resume your routine at a lower level, and gradually work back up. As a rule of thumb, take about as much time as you missed to get back up to where you were before.

A Word about Motivation

It only hurts for a little while; after that, if Senator William Proxmire is right, you'll "feel immortal." Until you get to that exalted place, however, you may have some resistance to lacing up your running shoes. Says Dr. Cooper:

> Much depends on your frame of mind. Make a resolution to stick with the program for eight weeks—and no weasling out of it. Once you're past that period, I can promise you that you'll begin to enjoy your workout. After eight to ten weeks, you sense the change. You'll find yourself looking forward to your exercise, longing for it as an accustomed pleasure.

Another aid is jogging with a partner. J. A. Archer, vice-president of Schlitz, who was running five miles a day at age 58, said, "Get a guy who will meet you at 6 A.M. on a cold day." With such a devoted partner you will be shamed into it. Remember, however, the purpose of jogging with someone else is companionship—not competition.

Others suggest getting the family into the act. If you have trouble finding a partner, contact the National Jogging Association, 1910 K Street, N.W., Suite 202, Washington, D.C. 20006; in other parts of the country, the National Roadrunners Association, 2737 Devonshire Place, N.W., Washington, D.C., 20008. They will let you know about jogging groups in your vicinity. (They are also an excellent source of information of any aspect of jogging.)

---

the world's oldest exercise: walking

It's the cheapest, the easiest, the most accessible, the least conspicuous, and maybe the best.

A brisk walk in the open air brings nearly every muscle into play. It is aerobic, if the pace is fast enough and the distance long enough.

The massaging action of the leg muscles on the veins improves the flow of blood back to the heart.

When you walk, keep your knees and ankles loose; point your toes straight ahead. Hold your chest and head high, back straight. Swing your legs directly forward from the hip joints. Don't shuffle—push your feet off the ground. Swing your shoulders and arms freely and easily. Breathe deeply.

Holding head erect and the back straight does not mean walking around with a stiff, military bearing. Your head should be free to turn.

Allow extra time to catch trains or get to meetings so you can walk. Take a walk just for the fun of it, especially when feeling tense or in need of a break in the routine. Enjoy your walking. Use it both for exercise and sight-seeing. Walk briskly if exercise is the primary motivation, but slow down from time to time to enjoy what is going on around you.

If it's records you're after, John Lees of Brighton, England, took less than two months to walk from City Hall in Los Angeles to City Hall in New York. Georgyi Bushuyev took 238 days to walk from Riga, Latvia, to Vladivostok, U.S.S.R. Georgyi was 50 at the time. And if it's the bizarre you're after, think of Mr. Plennie L. Wingo, a Texan who took eighteen months to cover the 8000 miles between Santa Monica, California, and Istanbul, Turkey: Mr. Wingo walked the entire distance backwards.

—————————— a basic jogging program ——————————

Here is a systematic aerobic regimen. Designed by the President's Council on Physical Fitness and Sports, it can be performed by most men and women of all ages. Those who are in good shape will find it easy and should proceed with a stepped-up routine. The program makes use of the principles of "interval training," which allows a greater amount of work to be performed in a shorter period of time. It alternates periods of high exertion, such as jogging, with recovery periods, during which less strenuous activity is performed.

The accompanying pace chart should be used to help anyone follow the basic jogging program provided below or any other exercise program that involves walking, jogging, or running. If the distance a person is walking, jogging, or running is known, timing over these distances will determine speed.

Pace	Speed mph	55 yds.	110 yds.	220 yds.	440 yds.	880 yds.	1 mile
				Time for Various Distances (Min:Sec)			
Slow walk	3	:38	1:15	2:30	5:00	10:00	20:00
Moderate walk	4	:28	:56	1:52	3:45	7:30	15:00
Fast walk	4.5	:25	:50	1:40	3:20	6:40	13:20
Slow jog	5	:22	:45	1:30	3:00	6:00	12:00
Moderate jog	6	:19	:38	1:15	2:30	5:00	10:00
Fast jog	7	:17	:33	1:05	2:09	4:17	8:34
Slow run	8	:15	:29	:57	1:54	3:47	7:34
Moderate run	9	:13	:25	:50	1:40	3:20	6:40
Fast run	10	:11	:22	:45	1:30	3:00	6:00
Competitive running	11	:10.5	:21	:41	1:22	2:44	5:27
	12	:9.5	:19	:38	1:15	2:30	5:00
	15	:7.5	:15	:30	1:00	2:00	4:00

Week 1

Day 1 Walk 880 yds.	(1/2 mile)	@ Slow pace with stretching		
Jog 55 yds.	(25 sec.)		Walk 55 yds.	2 times
Day 2 Walk 880 yds.	(1/2 mile)	Easy pace with stretching		
Jog 55 yds.	(25 sec.)		Walk 55 yds.	4 times
Day 3 Repeat Day 2				

Week 2

Day 1 Walk 440 yds.	(1/4 mile)	@ Moderate pace with stretching		
Jog 55 yds.	(25 sec.)		Walk 55 yds.	4 times
Walk 440 yds.	(1/4 mile)		Moderate pace	
Jog 110 yds.	(50 sec.)		Walk 110 yds.	
Day 2 Repeat Day 1				
Day 3 Walk 440 yds.	(1/4 mile)	@ Moderate pace with stretching		
Jog 55 yds.	(22 sec.)		Walk 55 yds.	4 times
Walk 220 yds.	@ Moderate pace			
Jog 110 yds.	(45 sec.)		Walk 110 yds.	2 times

Week 3

Day 1 Walk 440 yds.	(1/4 mile)	@ Moderate pace with stretching		
Jog 55 yds.	(22 sec.)		Walk 55 yds.	4 times
Jog 110 yds.	(45 sec.)		Walk 110 yds.	4 times
Day 2 Repeat Day 1				
Day 3 Walk 440 yds.		@ Moderate pace with stretching		
Jog 55 yds.	(22 sec.)		Walk 55 yds.	4 times
Walk 220 yds.	(1/8 mile)		Moderate pace	
Jog 220 yds.	(slow)		Walk 220 yds.	
Jog 110 yds.	(45 sec.)		Walk 110 yds.	2 times

Week 4

Day 1 Walk 440 yds.		@ Moderate pace with stretching		
Jog 55 yds.			Walk 55 yds.	4 times
Jog 110 yds.			Walk 110 yds.	4 times
Jog 220 yds.			Walk 220 yds.	
Day 2 Repeat Day 1				
Day 3 Walk 440 yds.		@ Moderate pace with stretching		
Jog 55 yds.			Walk 55 yds.	4 times
Jog 44 yds.	Slow pace		Walk 220 yds.	
Jog 110 yds.			Walk 110 yds.	3 times

Continued on following page.

Week 5

Day 1 Walk 440 yds.   @ Brisk pace with stretching
- Jog 110 yds.   Walk 110 yds.   2 times
- Jog 220 yds.   Walk 220 yds.   2 times
- Jog 330 yds.   Walk 330 yds.

Day 2 Repeat Day 1

Day 3 Walk 440 yds.   @ Brisk pace with stretching
- Jog 110 yds.   Walk 110 yds.   2 times
- Jog 440 yds.   Walk 440 yds.
- Jog 220 yds.   Walk 220 yds.   2 times

Week 6

Day 1 Walk 440 yds.   @ Brisk pace with stretching
- Jog 110 yds
- Jog 440 yds.   Walk 440 yds.
- Jog 55 yds.   (19 sec.)   Walk 55 yds.   4 times

Day 2 Repeat Day 1

Day 3 Walk 440 yds.   @ Brisk pace with stretching
- Jog 110 yds.   Walk 110 yds.   2 times
- Jog 880 yds.   Slowly
- Jog 55 yds.   (19 sec.)   Walk 55 yds.   4 times

Week 7

Day 1 Walk 440 yds.   @ Brisk pace with stretching
- Jog 110 yds.   Walk 110 yds.   4 times
- Jog 330 yds.   Walk 330 yds.
- Jog 220 yds.   Walk 220 yds.   3 times

Day 2 Repeat Day 1

Day 3 Walk 440 yds.   @ Brisk pace with stretching

Jog 1 mile slowly (vary pace and walk if necessary)
- Jog 55 yds.   Walk 55 yds.   4 times

Week 8

Day 1 Walk 440 yds.   @ Brisk pace with stretching
- Jog 110 yds.   Walk 110 yds.   3 times
- Jog 220 yds.   Walk 110 yds.   2 times
- Jog 440 yds.   Walk 440 yds.

Day 2 Repeat Day 1

Day 3 Walk 440 yds.   @ Brisk pace with stretching
- Jog 1 mile
- Jog 110 yds.   Walk 110 yds.   2 times

Week 9

Day 1 Walk 440 yds.   @ Brisk pace with stretching
- Jog 110 yds.   Walk 110 yds.   3 times
- Jog 330 yds.   Walk 110 yds.   2 times
- Jog 440 yds.   Walk 440 yds.

Day 2 Repeat Day 1

Day 3 Walk 440 yds.   @ Brisk pace with stretching
- Jog 220 yds.   Walk 110 yds.   2 times
- Jog 1 mile

Continued on following page.

Week 10

Day 1 Walk 440 yds.   @ Brisk pace with stretching
       Jog 110 yes.   Walk 110 yds.   4 times
       Jog 440 yds.   Walk 220 yds.
       Jog 220 yds.   Walk 220 yds.   2 times
Day 2 Repeat Day 1
Day 3 Walk 440 yds.   @ Brisk pace with stretching
       Jog 220 yds.   Walk 110 yds.   2 times
       Jog 1 mile
       Jog 55 yds.   Walk 55 yds.   2 times

Week 11

Day 1 Walk 440 yds.   @ Brisk pace with stretching
       Jog 110 yds.   Walk 55 yds.   4 times
       Jog 220 yds.   Walk 110 yds.   3 times
       Jog 440 yds.   Walk 220 yds.
Day 2 Repeat Day 1
Day 3 Walk 440 yds.   @ Brisk pace with stretching
       Jog 1½ miles (vary pace and walk if necessary)

Week 12

Day 1 Walk 440 yds.   @ Brisk pace with stretching
       Jog 220 yds.   Walk 110 yds.   2 times
       Jog 110 yds.   Walk 55 yds.   4 times
       Jog 440 yds.   Walk 220 yds.   2 times
Day 2 Walk 440 yds.   @ Brisk pace with stretching
       Jog 440 yds.   Walk 220 yds.   2 times
       Jog 330 yds.   Walk 110 yds.   2 times
       Jog 110 yds.   Walk 55 yds.   3 times
Day 3 Walk 440 yds.   @ Brisk pace with stretching
       Jog 1½ miles at your own pace
       Walk 440 yds.

Week 13

Day 1 Walk 440 yds.   @ Brisk pace with stretching
       Jog 220 yds.   Walk as necessary 3 times
       Jog 330 yds.   Walk as necessary 2 times
       Jog 440 yds.   Walk as necessary 2 times
Day 2 Walk 440 yds.   @ Brisk pace with stretching
       Jog 1½ miles—vary pace
       Walk 440 yds.
Day 3 Walk 440 yds.   @ Brisk pace with stretching
       Jog and walk when necessary for 2 miles
       Walk 440 yds.

Continued on following page.

Week 14

Day 1 Walk 440 yds.   @ Brisk pace with stretching
     Jog 440 yds.   Walk as necessary 2 times
     Jog 220 yds.   Walk as necessary 4 times
     Jog 880 yds.   Walk 220 yds.
Day 2 Walk 440 yds.   @ Brisk pace with stretching
     Jog 2 miles—vary pace, walk when necessary
     Walk 440 yds,
Day 3 Walk 440 yds.   @ Brisk pace with stretching
     Jog 880 yds.   Walk as necessary
     Jog 440 yds.   Walk as necessary 2 times
     Jog 220 yds.   Walk as necessary 4 times
     Walk 220 yds.

Week 15

Day 1 Walk 440 yds.   @ Brisk pace with stretching
     Jog 880 yds.   Walk as necessary 2 times
     Jog 220 yds.   Walk as necessary 4 times
     Jog 440 yds.
     Walk 220 yds.
Day 2 Walk 440 yds.   @ Brisk pace with stretching
     Jog 2 miles at your own pace
     Walk 220 yds.
Day 3 Same as Day 1

Week 16

Day 1 Walk 440 yds.   @ Brisk pace with stretching
     Jog 110 yds.   Walk as necessary 4 times
     Jog 220 yds.   Walk as necessary 4 times
     Jog 440 yds.   Walk as necessary 2 times
     Jog 880 yds.   Walk as necessary 2 times
     Walk 220 yds.
Day 2 Walk 440 yds.   @ Brisk pace with stretching
     Jog 20 minutes at own pace
     Walk 220 yds.
Day 3 Walk 440 yds.   @ Brisk pace with stretching
     Jog 24 minutes at own pace   Walk if necessary
     Walk 220 yds.

jogging do's and don'ts

If you are out of shape, start your aerobics with a week of walking briskly. This gives your heart time to get accustomed to new demands, and to loosen the muscles and tendons. In any given session, start off slowly after you have completed your warmup routine, and build to your desired level of exertion. "Avoid straining and pushing yourself to the extent that you become overly fatigued," says Dr. Cooper. "Such intense effort at the outset of an exercise program is not only dangerous, it also defeats your basic purpose. Instead of feeling more fit and more vigorous, you'll just feel chronically tired."

Cooling down after your aerobic program is as important as warming up to it (see next section). Those who come to a screeching halt, collapsing in an armchair as soon as their workout time is up, are likely to suffer dizzy spells, fainting, or something more serious. Ease up gradually, slowing down your pace over a five-minute period. If you have been jogging outdoors, slow down to a walk over a five-minute period and continue to walk for a while afterwards.

Dr. Cooper explains that during running most of the blood shifts to the legs. When the activity is suddenly halted, the blood stays in the legs, as the muscle do not help return the blood to the heart and the brain.

In addition to tapering down the level of exertion, remain at the same air temperature. Don't hop immediately into a hot room or shower; avoid steam rooms and saunas until you cool down. The sudden warmth will cause the capillary vessels to dilate, thus making it that more difficult to supply the heart and brain with blood.

Some experts advise doing calisthenics as you taper down from your aerobics, especially if your aerobics involve mainly the legs and not the arms and upper body. Push-ups, jumping jacks, or the exercises recommended below for warming up will do nicely.

how to jog

According to the President's Council on Physical Fitness, there is no one correct method of jogging. While methods do vary, here are some general guidelines:

Stand up straight, avoiding the tendency to lean. Keep your back as straight as you can without being uncomfortable. Keep the head up.

Hold your arms slightly away from your body. Bend them at the elbows so that the forearms are approximately parallel to the ground. Shaking and relaxing the arms and shoulders from time to time will help reduce tightness.

There are several acceptable techniques for how the foot hits the ground. One is to land first on the heel, slightly before the bottom of the foot touches ground; then rock forward, taking off from the ball of the foot for the next step. If this seems uncomfortable, try a more flat-footed style, landing on the entire bottom of the foot.

> *Don't land on the balls of the feet, as sprinters do, as it will create unnecessary foot and leg soreness.*
>
> *Keep your steps short, letting the foot strike the ground beneath the knee rather than reaching out to the front. The slower you run, the shorter your stride should be.*
>
> *Do not hold your breath. Breathe deeply with mouth open. Blow out hard. Periodically, take several deep breaths and blow out completely; this will aid muscle relaxation.*

The Hazards

Exercising can be hazardous if done carelessly, incorrectly, or in excess. The darkest onus, of course, is sudden heart attack. If, due to artery obstructions, the heart muscles are receiving an uneven supply of blood, the sudden demand of strenuous exercise may cause a spasm of fluttering or trembling instead of a regular beat. This is known as fibrillation, and is a common sort of heart attack.

As mentioned earlier, the stress-electrocardiogram is the best way to detect potential problems. Dr. George Sheehan, a New Jersey cardiologist who runs an hour a day, advises what he calls the "talk test" for those who stubbornly resist taking a physical. "If you can't hold a conversation while running because you're out of breath, then you're overdoing it," he says.

Foot and ankle difficulties are, according to Dr. Cooper, the most frequent problems among joggers. Our bodies were not built for running on hard surfaces. Pains in the muscles and joints are common; achilles tendonitis—inflammation of the large tendon that connects the calf and heel—occurs frequently, even among trained athletes; joggers's heel, caused by landing too hard on the heel, is common among beginners who hit the ground incorrectly.

For these reasons, running on cushiony surfaces, like grass or sand, is preferred. So is running over distance rather than running in place. If you do run in place, try to do it on a carpet, and keep your running shoes on.

Reportedly, the two most common problems among runners are inflammations of the knee, and shin splits (inflammations in the muscles and tendons between the lower leg bones). Such difficulties are also caused by running on uncushioned surfaces, from landing incorrectly, and from wearing improper shoes. In addition, running on unbanked tracks of small circumference will aggravate the ankles and knees. Dr. Cooper recommends avoiding tracks that require more than 25 laps to the mile.

how to avoid achilles heel

Achilles Stretch

Stand 2 or 3 feet from wall.
Lean against wall with outstretched arms.
Move left leg forward half a step.
Move right leg backward half a step.
Lower right heel to the floor.
Lean body toward wall to stretch right heel tendon.
Hold 5–10 counts, breathing normally.
Reverse leg positions and repeat 3–6 times for each leg.

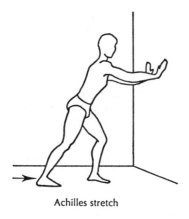

Achilles stretch

Chronic fatigue is reported by exercisers who overdo it. It is normal to be tired after a workout, but chronic fatigue indicates that you are going at a pace you are not ready for. If chronically tired, change your schedule to incorporate one resting day after every two days of exercise. Or, exercise at a lower rate for a longer time.

If you follow the guidelines provided throughout this chapter, most common hazards can be prevented. It is, however, vital that you remain alert for warning signs, some of which may indicate serious disorders. The following information is based on Dr. Lenore Zohman's guidelines for heeding your body's own signals.

danger signs

Signs	Possible causes
Abnormal heart action: irregular pulse palpitations in chest or throat sudden bursts of rapid heartbeat sudden very low pulse	Extra or reduced number of heart beats, or cardiac rhythm disorders. This may or may not be dangerous.
Pain in center of chest or in the arm or throat	Could be angina, but not necessarily.
Dizziness, lightheadedness, cold sweat, fainting immediately following exercise	Could be a sign of insufficient supply of blood to the brain.

In all of the above cases, *consult your physician before resuming your exercise program.* If any of the symptoms in category three occur, stop the exercise and lie down with your feet elevated, or put your head down between your legs until the symptoms pass. If chest pains occur during exercise, slow down to a gradual halt.

warning signs

Other signs may be handled on your own. If the symptoms persist, however see a physician.

Signs	Comments
Persistent rapid heart even after exercise ceases	You are probably overdoing it. Next time build up more slowly and level off at a lower heart rate.
Inflammation in the joints	If you have arthritis, gout, or other joint problems, use your customary remedies. Do not resume until condition subsides. Try better shoes, or softer surfaces, switch to swimming if it persists.

Signs	Comments
Nausea or vomiting after exercise	You are probably going too hard or cooling down too rapidly, preventing adequate oxygen from reaching the intestine.
Extreme breathlessness as long as ten minutes after exercising	You are overtaxing yourself—cut down the level of exertion.
Shin splints, usually noticed as pain on the front or sides of the lower leg	Muscles or connective tissues are inflamed.
Sudden onset of insomnia	You may be overdoing it. Excess fatigue can actually interfere with sleep.
Pain in the calf muscles	May be due to muscle cramps or poor circulation. Use thicker soles, warm up and cool down adequately. If that doesn't do it, you may have poor circulation—consider cycling or swimming.
Sticking feeling under the rib cage	Caused by a spasm of the diaphragm. Sit down, lean forward, attempting to push the abdominal organs up against the diaphragm.
Charley horse	You are out of shape and unaccustomed to exercise. Take a hot bath, and be sure to warm up properly next time. Be less strenuous too.
Blisters	Your shoes or socks don't fit.

What to Wear

Loose, comfortable clothing is considered the rule. You needn't wear one of those colorful jogging suits that are in vogue, but they are quite practical and comfortable. Purchasing one also provides the sort of psychological commitment that might make a difference when you need extra motivation.

Do not wear rubberized or plastic clothing. Some people are attracted to them because they raise the perspiration level, which they erroneously think will help them lose weight. What it can do is lead to excessive dehydration and salt loss, which in turn can lead to heat stroke or heat exhaustion because the sweat can't evaporate.

Make sure your shoes fit properly. The soles should be firm, the tops pliable, and they should have good arch supports. Ripple or crepe soles—particularly those made for long-distance running—are excellent, especially if you intend to jog on hard surfaces.

The beginner is advised not to use inexpensive sneakers, tennis shoes, or cross-country shoes without well-protected heels or arch support. Olympic Gold Medal winner Frank Shorter, who averages seventeen miles of running a day, advises, "Lay out around $25 right away to avoid injuries. If you quit, you'll still have a good pair of shoes to kick around in."

Your socks should be soft, heavy, and well-fitting. Thin socks under the heavy ones are recommended. Cotton absorbs perspiration, but does not insulate well against friction. Nylon offers the opposite. It's up to you. Try both and decide.

Where to Jog

One of the reasons jogging has become the biggest participatory sport in the United States is that it can be done almost anywhere. If possible, beginners should avoid hard surfaces such as cement or asphalt, at least for the first few weeks. Seek out a running track at your local high school or university; grass playing fields, dirt paths, parks, and golf courses are reasonably accessible to most people.

In inclement weather there is always the local YMCA, school or church gymnasium, parking garages, well-protected shopping centers, your basement, or even your living room or office.

To add spice to your jogging routine, vary your scenery and terrain. Remember to give the right of way to automobiles, bicycles, and dogs. And stay away from heavy traffic.

When to Jog

Almost any time of day will do, although joggers seem to prefer early morning when the air is clean and fresh, or late afternoon when they can work off the built-up tensions of the day. Don't jog during the first hour after eating—two hours if your meal was heavy—and don't jog in the middle of a hot, humid day. If the air pollution is bad, it may be wise to skip it that day. The same is true for extremely cold weather if you are new at it. Says Dr. William Hood, chief of cardiology at Boston

a businessman's cross-country health guide

City	Best Hotels for Health Facilities	Best Health Clubs*	Best for Walking or Jogging
Pittsburgh	Howard Johnson's Motor Lodge (in Chatham Center)	Pittsburgh Athletic Assn. (members and guests), Golden Triangle YMCA	Point Park State Park (once the sites of Fts. Duquesne and Pitt)
San Francisco		Ambassador Health Club Birt's Conditioning Clinic (in the Marine's Memorial Club)	Golden Gate Park or (for a climbing walk) to the top of Telegraph Hill
Seattle		Washington Athletic Club (members and guests)	University Arboretum (a 10-min. ride from downtown); best walk: along the colorful waterfront
Washington, D.C.	Watergate Hotel	WMCA	The Ellipse (behind the White House, between 15th and 17th Sts., N.W.); towpath of the C&O Canal

*Many of these cities have one or another of the chain health clubs, such as Vic Tanny's, Jack LaLanne, or President's Health Spas. YMCAs are also prevalent, and only noted here when they offer exceptional facilities for visiting executives.

a businessman's cross-country health guide

City	Best Hotels for Health Facilities	Best Health Clubs*	Best for Walking or Jogging
Atlanta	Howard Johnson's 57 Hotel	Downtown YMCA	Piedmont Park, 3 mi. north of downtown; Downtown YMCA, for indoor jogging
Boston	Sheraton-Boston Colonial Hilton, Wakefield (in the Rt. 128 area)	Boston YMCA (which caters to executives)	Boston Public Garden, Boston Common, both for walks; Charles River banks for jogs
Chicago	Sheraton-Chicago Continental Plaza	Chicago Health Clubs	Grant Park and the lakefront
Cleveland	Hollenden House	Downtown Businessmen's Health Club Central YMCA	Central YMCA for indoor jogging
Detroit	Detroit Hilton Somerset (in suburban Troy, Mich.)	Detroit Athletic Club Uptown Athletic Club (both private, available to guests of members)	Belle Isle, a $6 round-trip cab ride from downtown

Continued on following page.

City	Best Hotels for Health Facilities	Best Health Clubs*	Best for Walking or Jogging
Houston	Houston Oaks Hotel Holiday Inn (year-round pool)	Houston Club University Club (both with membership requirements)	Memorial Park Allen Park
Los Angeles	Century Plaza near ABC Entertainment Center, housing the fully equipped Century West Club	Beverly Hills Health Club for Men (there is a women's club, too)	Beaches near the city's west side and Santa Monica; Griffith Park for city joggers
New York	City Squire Motor Inn (indoor pool)	New York Athletic Club (tops for squash, but guest requirements strictly observed)	Central Park Reservoir (enter at 86th St.) is city's best for joggers
Philadelphia	Marriott Motor Hotel	Philadelphia Athletic Club (the usual membership rules obtain)	Rittenhouse Square (for pre-rush-hour jogs), Fairmount Park or walkways of Benjamin Franklin Pkwy. (for walkers)

Continued on following page.

City Hospital, "The circulatory stress combined with cold could trigger heart problems for the novice."

According to Dr. Cooper, the ideal exercise weather is 40 to 85 degrees F., with less than 60 percent humidity, and a wind velocity below 15 mph. If you are exercising outside the range of those limits, cut down the duration and intensity of your workout.

If the weather suddenly shifts to sizzling, slow down for at least two weeks and give your body a chance to adjust to the new conditions. Above 95 degrees, stop all strenuous exercise. Stop at 90 if the humidity is above 80 percent. In hot weather, drink lots of water, and increase your salt intake.

If you are physically fit, Dr. Hood's cold weather warning does not necessarily apply. But try to dress so that you'll sweat about as much as you would on a warm day. Keep your head and neckline open enough for heat to escape. Some wear headbands rather than hats to keep their ears warm.

Normally, air is warmed up by the time it gets to your chest. But if the temperature drops too far, too much icy air can rush into your windpipe, constricting the coronary arteries. Dr. Cooper advises wearing a loose-knit scarf over your mouth to help warm up the air.

Other cold-weather precautions include loosening up indoors, starting out more slowly, and always letting someone know where you will be exercising.

Dr. Hood says that "the noncardiac hazards of cold weather jogging are greatest." He advises switching to indoor exercise or his favorite substitute, cross-country skiing, to avoid "slippery roads, uneven footing, skidding cars, and poor visibility for drivers."

Stop at the first sign of chest pain. "That's a basic rule under any condition," says Dr. Cooper, "even more important when exercising in cold weather."

Speaking of cold, don't work out if you have one. "You should never exercise while you suffer from an acute infection," writes Dr. Cooper, "and a common cold is just that. Also stop exercising if you have the flu, an intestinal upset, or other virus disorders. If you have a fever, wait until your temperature returns to normal. Then wait at least an additional 24 hours."

exercises for warming up and cooling down

Each aerobic session should be preceded by a period of light warm-up exercises in order to gradually increase respiration, heart rate, and body temperature, and to stretch ligaments. This is especially important for people over 40.

The following warmup exercises are recommended by the President's Council on Physical Fitness. They may be performed by both men and women.

1. Bend and Stretch:

    Stand erect with your feet in line with your shoulders.
    Slowly, bend forward and down, with knees flexed, stretching gently in an attempt to touch your fingers to your toes.
    Return to starting position.
    Repeat 10 times.

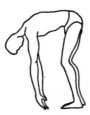

Flexed leg back stretch

2. Knee Lift:

    Stand erect, arms at sides, feet together.
    Raise your left knee as high as possible, grasping the leg with your hands and pulling the knee against the body. Keep your back straight throughout.
    Lower to starting position.
    Repeat with right leg.
    Perform 10 times with each leg.

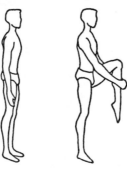

Knee lift

3. Wing Stretcher:
>   Stand erect with elbows at shoulder height.
>   Clench your fists in front of your chest, knuckles of each hand touching one another.
>   Vigorously thrust elbows backward without arching back.
>   Keep your head erect and your elbows at shoulder height throughout.
>   Return to starting position.
> Repeat 20 times.

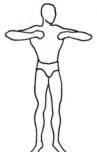

Wing stretcher

4. Half Knee-Bend:
>   Stand erect with hands on hips.
>   Bend knees halfway, while extending your arms forward; keep palms down.
>   Return to starting position.
> Repeat 10 times.

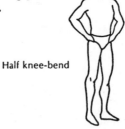
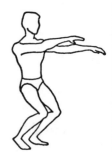

Half knee-bend

5. Arm Circles:
>   Stand erect with arms extended sideward at shoulder height; keep palms facing up.
>   Rotate hands in small circles backward.
>   Keep head erect throughout.
>   Repeat circles 15 times backward.
> Turn palms down, and describe 15 circles in the forward direction.

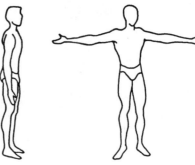

Arm circles

These warm-up exercises should all be done slowly. The point is to loosen up with them, not to get a workout. If the number of repetitions suggested here seems too strenuous, stop at the point where you begin to feel uncomfortable. If, on the other hand, they seem too easy, add on some repetitions; but avoid getting yourself exhausted. Since these are not aerobic, they will do little for your cardiovascular system. Therefore, save your energy for the conditioning session to follow. (These warm-up exercises can be done, of course, at times other than preceding aerobics; if you feel like loosening up while working in your office, this is a good way to do it without working up a sweat).

Lower Back Helpers

The following exercises are recommended by the President's Council for stretching the lower back area and helping to prevent lower back problems. Since most sedentary businessmen put a good deal of pressure on their lower backs, that is a common area of aches and pains when beginning an exercise program. You might add these to your warm-up program, or do them regularly as a back strengthener.

for your lower back

1. Standing Reach:
   Stand erect with feet in line with shoulders.
   Extend your arms directly overhead.
   Stretch as high as possible, keeping your heels on the ground.
   Hold for 15 to 30 seconds.

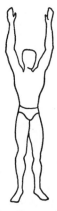

Standing reach

2. Flexed-Leg Back Stretch:
> Stand erect with feet in line with shoulders.
> Starting with arms at side, slowly bend forward.
> Keep the knees flexed.
> Touch the ground between the feet, or as close to it as is comfortable.
> Hold for 15 to 30 seconds.
> Repeat 2–3 times.

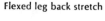

Flexed leg back stretch

3. Alternate Knee Pull:
> Lie on your back with your feet outstretched and your arms at your side.
> Pull your right leg to your chest.
> Grasp the knee with both arms and hold for 5 seconds.
> Repeat with the left leg.
> Perform with each leg 7–10 times.

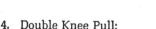

Alternate knee pull

4. Double Knee Pull:
> Lie on your back with your feet outstretched and your hands at your sides.
> Pull both legs to your chest.
> Lock your arms around your legs.
> Pull your buttocks slightly off the ground.
> Hold for 20–40 seconds.
> Repeat 7–10 times.

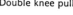

Double knee pull

5. Torso Twist:
> Lie on your back with your knees bent and your feet on the ground.
> Secure your feet under a heavy chair, or some other object, to prevent them from lifting (this is optional but preferred).

Lace your fingers behind your neck.
Curl your torso into the upright position and twist, touching your right elbow to your left knee.
Return to starting position.
Repeat, twisting in the opposite direction.
Exhale coming up, inhale going down.
Repeat series 5–15 times.

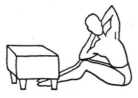

indoor exercising

If you are pressed for time, if the weather is foul, or if you abhor the idea of having the neighbors see you huff and puff, you might want to do your exercising indoors. Here are some tips for making the most of your home or office:

> *Running in place is an acceptable—if temporary—compromise, if you get your heart to pound at the requisite rate. It can be harmful to the ankles, however. Put on some rousing music at the right tempo for your rate of exercise; you will naturally fall into step.*
> *Dr. Cooper recommends adding variety to indoor jogging, by utilizing a sturdy set of three steps. Run up and down, turning at the top and bottom so that you always face forward. At a rate of twenty complete trips a minute, it is the equivalent, Cooper says, to stationary running at 80–90 steps per minute.*
> *You can also use one step—a footstool properly anchored will do. Start with both feet on the floor, step up with one, then bring the other up. Then return both feet to the floor, one after the other (don't jump). Do it rapidly, 30–40 full cycles per minute.*

Stationary Bicycles

These range from low-cost models ($25–35) to deluxe models at about $900 with built-in heart-rate monitors and simulated hills and valleys. The former are judged virtually worthless in an aerobic program, the latter are felt to be ideal for health clubs and YMCAs, but not necessary, and too expensive, for the home. In between are moderately priced models that offer just what you need for a home aerobic program: speed and mileage indicators and calibrated brake resistance devices that allow you to adjust to the desired level of work.

Treadmills

These too range widely, from about $100 to over $3000. The cheaper models are difficult to use effectively because they are muscle powered and seldom provide an incline. Some in the $400 range are motor driven and can be elevated by placing blocks under the front end. They only go up to 5 mph, however, enough for a slow jog.

In the $1000 to $1500 price range are the best machines for home use. They go up to 7–8 mph and have adjustable inclines. The type you will find in a laboratory are, of course the very best, but they are over $3500–hardly necessary for the home.

Using the treadmill requires adjusting speed and incline to the appropriate rates for your target zone. If you purchase one, seek professional guidance for its use.

Dr. Cooper observes that "many people who purchase expensive exercise equipment use it for only a short time and then store it, evidently preferring outdoor exercise (or no exercise at all)." It might be a lot cheaper, and more fun, to purchase a good pair of running shoes or a jump rope.

yoga exercises

The science of yoga dates back thousands of years to its roots in ancient India. As with other imports, it has suffered in the West from improper translations and misconceptions. A growing number of professionals have discovered that yoga (the branch of yoga associated with exercises is called "hatha yoga") is a system of proven exercises designed for reducing muscular tension and fostering the proper functioning of all bodily systems.

Unlike the exercises we have been discussing up to now, yoga exercises *are not muscle builders;* they are conditioners that increase muscle *tone* and flexibility. They are meant to be performed with no exertion, to conserve energy rather than use it up. Particularly good for sedentary businessmen, the exercises will stimulate circulation, and remove free-floating tension.

They will also help firm up muscle tone, straighten out backs that bend over desks all day, and loosen various joints, making the body more flexible and resilient. In addition, many yoga experts claim that they give a valuable internal message to vital organs such as the heart, liver, kidneys, stomach, and pancreas. They are also said to aid the functioning of the nervous and endocrine systems.

how to do yoga exercises

Never strain and never force your body into any position that is uncomfortable or painful. This is an extremely important point that is hazardous to ignore. We are used to exercises whose function is to make us work hard. That is fine for some purposes but not for yoga. Indeed, the very word "exercise" is misleading. In India, they are called asanas, *which translates better as postures or positions.*

The postures should be assumed slowly, gently, and easily. Never try to stretch or bend beyond your capability. As they are illustrated, the postures will be impossible for you to duplicate. Simply move slowly in the direction of the final posture and stop when you begin to feel a strain. Hold at that point. Pushing yourself will be self-defeating, and might result in a pulled muscle. Flexibility will grow over time.

Do the postures on a well-carpeted floor, with a clean blanket or sheet under you.

Dress in loose clothing. If you can't change into a comfortable outfit, loosen binding garments—ties, belts, bras, tight skirts, etc.

The room should be well ventilated, and spacious enough so that you can bend and stretch without interference.

a short yoga program

1. *The Back Stretch* This is an excellent warm-up, and if done gently will greatly help to limber your back and improve flexibility and posture.

As with all Yoga exercises, movements should be easy and graceful—never sudden. If your legs' tendons are tight, don't try to force them to stretch; if pain appears, ease up.

Sit erect with legs apart.
Pull right heel to groin and position sole of foot against left thigh.
With back straight, raise arms high above head.
Bend forward from the waist, keeping spine straight at first, and grasp toes with both hands. If you cannot reach that far easily, grasp ankle or calf, but do not allow left leg to bend at the knee.
Slowly curl the spine further foreward to touch your forehead to the left knee. Go as far as you can without straining (as in the fourth figure).
Return to an erect position. Straighten right leg, tuck left heel against groin and thigh, and repeat for the other side.

This sequence can be repeated for both legs if you like. Be sure not to bend suddenly, since the "stretch reflex" will automatically contract the large muscles behind your leg and prevent full flexing.

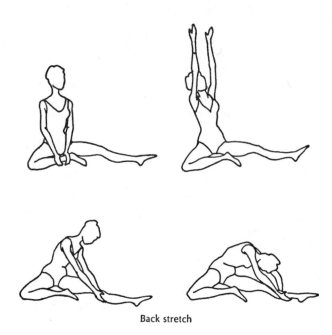

Back stretch

2. *The Shoulder Stand*   This posture will improve circulation, stimulate the thyroid gland, relax the leg muscles, and bring more blood to the upper regions of the body, especially to the brain.

Be very careful with this posture and the one following it; placing too much pressure on the neck can cause injury. The weight should be on your shoulders, upper back, and arms, *not the head or neck.*

Lie flat with your arms at your sides.

*Brace your palms against the floor, stiffen your abdomen and leg mus-
cles, and slowly raise your legs, knees straight.*

*When your legs are perpendicular to the floor, swing them back so
your hips leave the floor. Brace your hands against your hips for
support.*

*Slowly and carefully straighten to a modified upright position. At
first, remain in the position illustrated in the second figure. After
some weeks, if comfortable, straighten up still further, as in the
last picture.*

*Hold for about half a minute (advanced students of yoga often remain
in the position for as long as three to ten minutes), longer as you
progress. Keep legs relaxed.*

Return to the original position carefully, as follows:

Bend your knees and lower them to your forehead.

Place your hands at your sides for support.

Roll forward slowly and carefully.
When your buttocks touch the floor, straighten your legs.
Lower your legs to the floor.
Rest for a while.

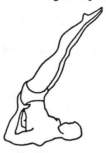

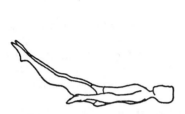

Since it is beneficial to invert the body from time to time, you should do it at least partially, even if you have difficulty with the shoulder stand. Raise your legs and hold them perpendicular to the body for a minute or so if you can't get your hips off the ground. Another alternative is to purchase a slant board. Specialty shops usually carry them for around $50. They are equipped with straps or bars under which you hook your feet for easy reclining at about a 45-degree angle.

Some books recommend the familiar head stand. However, unless done under the supervision of a bona fide yoga master, it can be dangerous, for it places great pressure on the blood vessels feeding the brain, and can easily strain the neck.

3. *The Plough* You may go into this from the shoulder stand, or begin anew after coming down from the shoulder stand.

Begin as you did the shoulder stand.
After swinging the legs back, let them fall very slowly toward the ground behind your head. Be very careful. If you let the legs come crashing down, or if you stretch further than your back muscles are prepared for, you can injure yourself.
In the complete posture, your toes should rest on the floor.
Keep knees straight, and chin tucked into the chest.
If you start to feel some strain as your legs descend, stop, let the legs hang, and hold.
Hold your maximum position for ten seconds at most.
Return to original position exactly as you did in the shoulder stand.
Rest afterward.

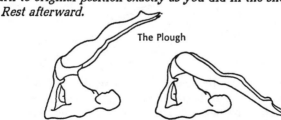

The Plough

4. *The Cobra*   This should greatly relax the upper back and neck
It is particularly pleasant after leaning over a desk all day.

Lie face down with your arms beneath the shoulders and your fore-
head on the floor.
Slowly, tilt your head backward.
Start by using the muscles of the lower back, not the arms. It is not
a push-up.
Keeping your eyes open, pretend you are trying to see behind you as
far as you can, rolling your head back, then your neck, shoulders,
and back. You should be able to feel each successive vertebra on
the spine being flexed.
Final position has arms slightly bent, spine arched, legs relaxed.
Hold about ten seconds.
Slowly reverse, lowering first your trunk, shoulders, neck, and head
until forehead rests on floor.
Repeat, if you like, after a brief pause.

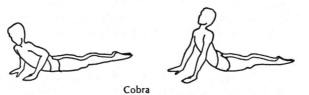

Cobra

5. *The Locust*   Do immediately following cobra.
Rest your chin on the mat.
Place hands at your sides (some advise making a fist; others advise
placing hands under the thighs).
Push hard against the floor and raise your legs, knees straight.
Hold about five seconds (less if it is a strain).
Slowly lower the legs. Repeat if you wish.
Rest with your cheek on the floor.

The Locust

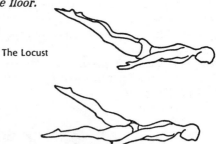

If you can only raise the legs an inch or so, that is fine. After a
short while, your body will become accustomed to this new posture
and the legs will raise higher. If you cannot raise them without a great
strain, do it one leg at a time until you can do it with both legs.

6. *The Twist*   This is excellent for providing relief from stiffness and tension in the spine. Note the positions carefully; it is often confusing at first. Be sure to twist in the right direction.

Cross your left leg over the outstretched right leg.
Cross your right arm over your left knee and grasp the right leg
    around the knee area.
Place your left hand on the floor behind you.
Slowly and easily twist your head and trunk to the left.
Hold at the maximum twist for about ten seconds.
Slowly return to the original position.
Repeat, reversing directions, twisting to the right, as pictured in the
    last drawing. Simply substitute right for left and vice versa in the
    instructions.

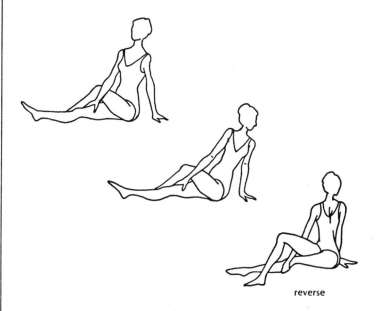

reverse

7. *The Rest Pose*   This is one of the most pleasant postures, and certainly the easiest. Do it at the end of your yoga session.

Lie on your back, hands at sides, palms up.
Close your eyes.
Allow the body to go limp.
Authorities differ as to what your mind should be doing at this time.
    Some advise just letting it be easy, not directing it in any way.
    Others advise intentionally relaxing muscle groups in order from
    the toes up the legs, torso, and head.
Remain supine for about thirty seconds.

————— **recommended reading: chapter 6** —————

Adult Physical Fitness, U.S. Government Printing Office, Washington, D.C. 20402.

Beyond Diet: Exercise Your Way to Fitness and Heart Health, Lenore Zohman. Pamphlet, free from Mazola Nutrition Information Service; Dept. ZD-NYT, Box 307, Conventry, Conn. 06238.

Exercise in the Office, Robert R. Spackman (Carbondale, Ill.: Southern Illinois University Press, 1968).

Introduction to Yoga, Richard Hittleman (New York: Bantam, 1969).

Royal Canadian Air Force Exercise Plans For Physical Fitness (New York: Pocket Books, 1972).

Running For Health and Beauty: A Complete Guide For Women, Kathryn Lance (New York: Bobbs-Merrill, 1977).

The Complete Book of Running, James F. Fixx (New York: Random House, 1977).

The New Aerobics, Kenneth Cooper (New York: Evans & Co., 1970).

The Perfect Exercise, Curtis Mitchell (New York: Simon & Schuster, 1976).

food
nutrition and
health

---

self-evaluation: your diet

1. Have you ever been put on a restricted diet?
    If so, do you often cheat?
2. Do you have a history of indigestion?
    Constipation?
    Diarrhea?
    Excessive flatulence?
3. Are you seriously overweight?
    Have you had difficulty losing weight?
    Do you gain easily?
4. Do you have insatiable cravings for food you know you should
    either limit or avoid entirely?
5. Do you salt your foods heavily?
6. Do you have sugar cravings?
    Do you give in to them frequently?
7. Do you eat a lot of fatty, high-cholesterol foods?
8. Do you feel particularly heavy and dull after most meals?
9. Do you often skip meals due to overwork?
10. Do you usually have a few drinks before or during meals?
11. Do you often "eat on the run"?
12. Do you eat while working?
13. Do you chew and swallow rapidly?
14. Are most of your lunches business lunches?
15. Do you occasionally lose your appetite due to tension?
16. Do you wake up hungry during the night?
    Do you wake up with indigestion during the night?
17. Does your energy level fluctuate excessively?
    Do you perk up immediately after eating only to slump soon
    afterward?

18. Do you get hyperactive, irritable, or disoriented if you go too long without eating?
19. Do you neglect to read the labels on packaged foods?
20. Do you eat a good deal of prepared, canned, or frozen foods?
21. Do you drink coffee? How much per day?

Yes answers to the above questions indicate possibly faulty nutrition habits. Pay particular attention to the information in this chapter relating to those questions. To help you evaluate your diet, keep a chart for two typical weeks. Make special note of your use of sugar, salt, caffeine, and high-cholesterol foods.

Date

Breakfast (note time)

Food   Drink

Snacks (note time)

Food   Drink

Lunch (note time)

Food   Drink

Snacks (note time)

Food   Drink

Supper (note time)

Food   Drink

Snacks (note time)

Food   Drink

Your foods shall be your remedies, and your remedies shall be your foods.
——Hippocrates

Despite the fact that the Hippocratic Oath is still recited by graduates of medical schools, the Greek physician's injunction about food is rarely heeded. An American Medical Association survey found that "medical education and medical practice have not kept abreast of the tremendous advances in nutritional knowledge and that there is inadequate recognition, support, and attention given to this subject in medical schools."

Nutrition is not a required subject in most medical schools, and where it is taught, it is scantily treated. Said Jean Mayer, professor of nutrition at Harvard, "Our studies at Harvard among residents suggest that the average physician knows a little more about nutrition than the average secretary—unless the secretary has a weight problem. Then she probably knows more than the average physician."

Experts have been increasingly critical of the typical American diet since World War II, when we began a wholesale move away from staples toward synthetic and highly processed items. We now eat between 21 and 25 percent fewer dairy products, vegetables, and fruits than we did 20 years ago.

While dissatisfaction is the rule, there is little agreement on precisely what we should and should not eat. One has to wade through a flood of conflicting opinions, controversies, and disputes. Says William Darby, president of the Nutritional Foundation in New York, quoted in *Time* magazine's excellent article, "Diet Crazes" (December 19, 1977): "The public has been inundated with claims and counterclaims by persons who are knowledgeable about nutrition, as well as by people who are not. So they're quite confused."

---

a national diet?

Congress has recently taken steps toward formulating a national nutritional policy. The Senate Committee on Nutrition and Human Needs, chaired by Senator George McGovern, recently recommended that HEW spend a "specific amount" yearly on introducing clinical nutrition training into the curriculum of every medical school by 1980. The committee also recommended that we:
1. reduce fat and cholesterol consumption
2. reduce sugar consumption
3. reduce salt consumption
4. increase consumption of fruits, vegetables, and whole grains
5. decrease consumption of meat, favoring poultry and fish

---

the cholesterol controversy

Cholesterol and triglyceride—the two principal fats in the bloodstream —are both closely associated with atherosclerosis and heart attack.

When abnormally high, the fats act as an irritant to artery walls, particularly to damaged ones, and contribute to the formation of plaques. It has been assumed that high amounts of *diet* cholesterol would elevate the level of *blood* cholesterol, and raise the risk of atherosclerosis. This has not actually been proved.

A good deal of controversy has developed around cholesterol and diet. Some would eliminate fats and cholesterol entirely, while others feel that eggs and other food items that allegedly provoke heart disease are nutritious and harmless if one has healthy digestion and a well-balanced vitamin intake. Most experts take the middle-of-the-road stance. The McGovern report, for example, recommends decreasing overall fat consumption from its present rate of approximately 40 percent of calorie intake to 30 percent, and cholesterol intake from its current 600–750 mg. a day to 300.

In the following sections, we will review both camps—first, the strong anti-diet-cholesterol approach, and then the counter-arguments.

The Longevity Center

The champion of the anti-cholesterol camp is Nathan Pritikin, an engineer and self-educated nutritionist who directs the Longevity Center in Santa Barbara, California, where diet and exercise are used to treat patients with degenerative diseases, including cardiovascular disorders.

Pritikin believes that 90 percent of heart disease can be prevented by a change to a low fat/low cholesterol diet. "This nonsense [cardiovascular disease] can all be stopped by a very moderate change in life-style," he states with conviction. "Medical costs can be decreased, and doctors can do useful things—practice prevention instead of crisis medicine."

Pritikin claims that patients on his diet have actually reversed the artery-obstructing process, which had been long considered impossible. Pritikin recalls being laughed at when his first announcements of reversal were made. Subsequently, more and more doctors concurred; the possibility of reversal is now gaining acceptance, although much reservation remains and few will go out on a limb for any particular method of treatment.

Dr. David Blankerhorn, who is investigating the effects of diet on atherosclerosis at the University of Southern California, admits to being "wildly excited" by his preliminary findings, which have recorded reversal in some patients on low-fat diets. Yet he remains guarded. "All we can say at this point," he acknowledges, "is that atherosclerosis can be reversed in humans."

Pritikin believes that even standard low-fat diets are too permissive. At the Longevity Center, those with serious problems are put on the "regression diet," whose allowance of fat and cholesterol is radically lower than the Senate Committee's recommendations.

Diet	% Fat	% Protein	% Carbohydrate	Cholesterol
Average American	40–45%	15–20%	40–45% (mostly refined)	600–750 mg/day
Longevity center	5–10%	10–15%	80% (entirely complex)	5 mg/day

Even the "maintenance diet," given to successful center graduates and recommended to everyone as the ideal preventive regimen allows only 100 mg. of cholesterol a day. In addition, it contains a host of other do's and don'ts (which skeptics feel may be more significant than the fat and cholesterol limitations that have attracted all the attention).

Pritikin's "2001 diet"

Do's

Dont's

Fruit and vegetable juices or water can be used instead of oils in cooking.

No butter, lard, oil or margarine. No cooking oil, salad oil.

Chicken, turkey, fish—no skin, trim all the fat off. Bake, broil, or roast.

No marbled or fatty meats, no organ meats (liver, kidneys, etc.); no animal skin, shellfish, or fatty fish; no duck or goose, lamb, pork, bacon, hot dogs, etc.

Only dairy products made from skimmed milk. Egg whites are permissible. Nonfat milk, not low fat.

No whole milk, creams, flavored yogurt, no cheeses made from whole milk, no non-dairy cream substitutes. No egg yolks.

All fruits and vegetables, raw, baked, or boiled (or sauteed in water). Limit dried fruits.

No avocados, nuts, or olives. No canned vegetables or fruit if sugar or additives are added. Avoid frozen foods in sauces. Most canned soups have fat and additives; so do bouillon cubes—avoid them.

Do's	Dont's
Whole grain breads, sourdough, tortillas, pita, matzos. Rolled oats and other whole grain cereals. Rice, noodles (preferably whole wheat).	None of those if baked with shortening or sugar. No cakes, crackers, sweet rolls, baking mixes with dried eggs and whole milk. No egg or spinach noodles.
Decaffeinated beverages, herb teas, no more than two ounces of alcohol a day.	No coffee, tea, sugar (watch for ingredients on packages), no salt (watch ingredients and add none). No sugared drinks, ice cream, pudding, etc.

When the center opened in 1976, after Pritikin had announced the results of preliminary studies showing reversal of artery closures, careful records were kept. A year later, the records were analyzed, and they indicated remarkable success.

Of the first 241 patients, 132 had angina, 98 had hypertension, 78 had had heart attacks (21 had at least two) and 30 had had bypass surgery. Arthritis, gout, diabetes, and other degenerative diseases were also common. At the end of the four-week program, the average blood cholesterol count decreased by 25 percent, triglyceride levels dropped an average of 40 percent, almost 90 percent of the hypertensives who had been on medication had normal blood pressure, overweight patients lost an average of ten pounds, and most smokers had stopped.

National exposure came to the Longevity Center when it became known that heart patients who had been told they needed coronary bypass surgery were treated there instead. Says Pritikin: "Of the candidates for bypass surgery who were admitted to the center from January 1976 to December 1976, virtually all improved to the degree that they no longer required surgery. Included in this group were a number whose vein grafts (from previous surgery) had closed." He is so confident that his procedures are an alternative to bypass operations that he states unequivocally, "We can guarantee 90 percent success. We've had 100 percent, but I'm only saying 90."

the longevity center

Located in Santa Barbara, California. Accommodations are comfortable, including swimming pools, golf courses, tennis courts, museums, and other recreational attractions.

Center staff consists of six physicians (two cardiologists), plus trained cooks and paramedics. Entering patients receive a comprehensive medical exam, including treadmill and resting electrocardiograms; 24-hour EKG monitoring (an ambulatory EKG) is available. Tests are given at the end of the stay, as well as during the four weeks, when necessary.

Blood pressure and weight are taken daily, blood tests weekly, and the patient visits a physician at least three times a week.

All meals are at the center: eight meals a day. Most meals consist of only an item or two. Though bland, veterans develop a liking for it.

The exercise program, taken mainly after meals, consists almost exclusively of walking (jogging or treadmill exercise are sometimes prescribed). Each patient's daily exercise chart is monitored by an exercise supervisor and medical staff.

One or two lecture-seminars are held every day on medical disorders, food composition, and exercise. Patients are instructed in cooking and shopping procedures so they can continue the regimen at home. They learn, for example, to cook without oil, sugar, salt, or eggs.

There are between 75 and 100 patients at the center; new groups begin weekly. The cost for the 26-day stay, including accommodations, meals, and medical expenses, is $4220 (plus any medical expenses above $1100). To encourage spouses to learn about the program a nominal charge of $780 is added for non-patient companions.

For information, contact Longevity Center, 1121 East Cabrillo Boulevard, Santa Barbara, Calif. 93103. Dr. Don Mannerberg is medical director. Telephone: (805) 966-3967.

The Counter-Arguments

Few can dispute the success of Pritikin's program. But it is not absolutely certain that the low fat diet is solely—or even primarily—responsible for that success, and, if it is, whether reversal of atherosclerosis is the reason. For one thing, critics note, the other dietary changes may also be significant. In addition, the patients are on an all-day regimen, with something scheduled virtually every minute. Programmed exercise routines, medical attention, and a full program of lectures and seminars are important parts of the four-week stay. How much do these other factors contribute to the center's success?

According to Pritikin, very little. He calls exercise "indispensable," but feels that even without it, the diet alone would do the trick. "Jogging without a change in diet," he maintains, "is worthless. If the arteries keep clogging because of eating fats, they will clog faster than jogging can increase circulation."

Pritikin points out that success has been achieved by people who simply follow the diet/exercise program and keep in touch by telephone.

Not everyone buys Pritikin's interpretation of his success. Cardiologist Meyer Friedman and psychologist Carl Thoresen, for example, feel that modification of behavior is, perhaps unknowingly, at least partially responsible. Others have postulated that the educational seminars—which some have labeled "evangelical"—are more significant than Pritikin admits. Teaching people to live healthy lives, combined with the other features of the program, may go a long way toward helping them cut down on other risk factors, such as smoking and drinking. According to one graduate, the program works 50 percent because of the diet, and 50 percent because of attitude.

Dr. Richard Passwater feels that "what makes these programs work is the fact that the diets are weight-loss diets, rich in micronutrients, and the regimens include adequate exercise, smoking restriction, and blood pressure control." He is not the only one to suggest that the real value of low cholesterol/low fat diets is not in lowering serum cholesterol, but in weight loss, which is certainly a major factor in heart disease.

Is Diet Cholesterol Really Bad?

Many experts believe that diet cholesterol is the culprit. Some epidemiological surveys indicate that populations with low fat/low cholesterol diets have less heart disease, but other factors are involved. To suggest that the low incidence of heart disease in primitive societies is due to low fat/low cholesterol diets ignores the fact that culture, genetics, and exercise might also play significant roles. To say that the reason Japanese emigrants to the United States had a higher incidence of heart disease than those who remained in Japan is because they increased dietary fat and cholesterol is to ignore the fact that pace of life, culture, behavior, and environment all changed too.

---

studies refuting the diet cholesterol theories

Diet cholesterol levels are almost identical for men and women, yet men have more heart attacks.
Americans, Swedes, and Britons consume nearly identical percentages of total fat, yet the death rate from coronary heart disease in the

United States is three times as high as in Sweden and twice as high as in Great Britain.

Exercise seems to reduce the level of blood cholesterol even when the diet remains the same.

Finns eat the same amount of fat and cholesterol as the Dutch, but have 2 1/2 times the amount of heart disease. Finns in the east of Finland have twice as many heart attacks as their countrymen in the west, but eat the same amount of fat.

Irish immigrants, in Boston for a decade, were compared with their brothers who remained in Ireland. The Americans ate nearly 500 calories a day less and about half the amount of butter and eggs, yet the brothers that remained in Ireland weighed 15 percent less, had lower blood cholesterol levels, and only half the incidence of high blood pressure.

The American diet has remained about the same with respect to cholesterol and fat since 1910, yet the rate of heart disease has increased 500 percent.

The Masai of Africa, who live almost entirely on meat and milk, were virtually free of coronary artery disease and hypertension. Their blood cholesterol levels were an amazing 120/100. Similar findings were made on Navajos in North America.

In other words, not everyone who eats a lot of fat and cholesterol gets atherosclerosis. Nor does everyone who has a heart attack have an abnormally high cholesterol count.

The Necessity of Cholesterol

Despite its negative image, cholesterol is an important substance in every body cell. It is a constituent of pituitary, adrenal, and gonadal hormones, it acts as a conductor of nerve impulses, and, as a constituent of bile, it helps to emulsify fats.

Writes Dr. Richard Passwater, an opponent of low cholesterol diets: "The healthy body closely regulates the production of cholesterol so that when we eat more cholesterol, the body produces less cholesterol to keep the amount of cholesterol available in the body constant. Likewise, if we eat less cholesterol, we make more."

Furthermore, the plaques that form on artery walls and obstruct blood flow are not made entirely of cholesterol—they contain fibrin, collagen protein, minerals, triglycerides, and phospholipids. In fact, some say that the earliest deposits contain no cholesterol at all.

The most recent findings indicate that cholesterol does not exist in the bloodstream as a single entity, but is transported as a component of carriers called "lipoproteins." One is called Low Density Lipoprotein (LDL), the other is called High Density Lipoprotein (HDL). More than the total amount of cholesterol, the ratio of HDL to LDL is now considered the key risk factor. Even if your total cholesterol level is high, you may have very little risk of heart disease if your HDL-LDL ratio is high (the higher the better).

Such findings have led many scientists away from diet-conscious colleagues. Dr. William B. Kannel, director of the famous Framingham Study (which isolated *blood* cholesterol as one risk factor in heart disease), concluded in his final report that there is "no discernible association between the amount of cholesterol in the diet and the level of cholesterol in the blood. No matter how much or how little animal fat there is in the diet, some people will have low levels of cholesterol in their blood; others will have moderate levels and others high levels."

What determines the level of blood cholesterol? No one is sure: it may have to do with hereditary tendencies, exercise levels, dietary factors such as the consumption of vitamin E or C, or even digestive problems. Some say that neural and hormonal imbalances will increase an overly stressed individual's improper assimilation of heavy foods, thus creating more blood fat and cholesterol than desirable.

Conclusions—If Any

What is the bottom line on the cholesterol controversy? Few would argue that cholesterol count is one risk factor, but most would be reluctant to single it out above cigarette smoking, exercise, emotional stress, heredity, or other variables. The National Heart and Lung Institute sums up the uncertainty:

> Although there is some evidence to support the popular belief that blood lipids (i.e. blood fats and cholesterol) are causally related to arteriosclerosis, and that a decrease in total and saturated fats in diet may help to prevent ... heart attack and stroke, the evidence is scientifically not entirely convincing. Therefore, recommendations concerning diet are based on personal impressions and fragmentary evidence rather than on scientific proof.

Yet, everyone agrees that Americans eat entirely too much fat and cholesterol. It makes us overweight, if nothing else. Further, it almost certainly *aggravates* atherosclerosis, even if it doesn't cause it.

Those with suspected heart problems, or who agree intuitively with theories blaming heart disease on cholesterol intake, might do well to follow Pritikin's regimen, or something close to it.* Others might want to cut down to the limits recommended by the more moderate Senate committee.

---

*Anyone with angina or other indications of heart condition should eat exactly what their doctors advise.

Type of Food	Cholesterol (mg. per oz.)	Fat (g. per oz.)
A. *Meats (lean)*		
Pork	24	7
Beef	27	6
Lamb	20	6
Veal	30	3
Organs (e.g., liver)	91	1
B. *Most fish*	24	2
C. *Shellfish*		
Crab	42	0.5
Lobster	66	0.5
Clams	50	0.5
Shrimp	50	0.5
D. *Fowl*		
(Chicken & turkey)	20	1
E. *Dairy Products*		
Whole milk	3	1.5
Low-fat (2%) milk	2	1
Skim milk	0	0
Buttermilk	0	0
Cream	34	14
Butter	83	24
Cottage cheese (uncreamed)	1	0.5
F. *Egg (1 whole)*	275	6
G. *Vegetables*	0	0.2
H. *Fruits*	0	0.1
I. *Nuts*	0	18
J. *Cereals*		
Breakfast cereals	0	0
Bread	10	1
Cake	25	5
Cookies	35	7
Waffles	55	4

a low cholesterol diet

Food	Total Daily No. of Ounces	Cholesterol	Fat
2 servings of fish, fowl, or lean meat	10	240 mg	70 grams
4 servings of vegetables	16	0	3
2 servings of salad with 2 tablespoons of oil dressing	8	0	30
2 glasses of skim milk	16	0	0
2 slices of bread	2	20	4.4
Oleomargarine	2	0	53
Fruit	6	0	0
One serving of cereal	2	0	1
Total for a day	62	260	158.4

trimming down

"Let me have men about me that are fat," implored Shakespeare's Julius Caesar, fearing the "lean and hungry look" of men like Cassius. Caesar would have little to worry about in most offices today. Despite a two-decade obsession with overweight, Americans are fatter than ever, according to a report from the National Center for Health Statistics in Washington. Fifteen years ago, the average American man weighed 166; now he is 172. That's a four percent weight gain, and it is paralleled in women, who have gone from 140 to 143. With one exception, every category of height and age has increased its average weight, sometimes as much as 14 pounds.

Weight and stress form a vicious cycle: overeating and poor digestion can result from stress; susceptibility to stress disorders increases with overweight. If you are 25 percent overweight your chances of having a heart attack are about 2 1/2 times greater. An overweight person is forcing the heart to pump nourishment to an abnormal quantity of tissue. The resulting wear and tear on your heart and blood vessels is tremendous, raising the risk of stroke, diabetes, hypertension, and heart disease.

Height-weight charts, of course, do not take into account differences in the body fat, musculature, hormonal balance, and metabolism.

recommended weights by body frame types

| Height | | Men | | | |
Feet	Inches	Small Frame	Medium Frame	Large Frame	Actual Average
5	2	112–120	118–129	126–141	
5	3	115–123	121–133	129–144	
5	4	118–126	124–136	132–148	
5	5	121–129	127–139	135–152	
5	6	124–133	130–143	138–156	160
5	7	128–137	134–147	142–161	
5	8	132–141	138–152	147–166	169.6
5	9	136–145	145–156	151–170	
5	10	140–150	146–160	155–174	178.8
5	11	144–154	150–165	159–179	
6	0	148–158	154–170	164–184	188.5
6	1	152–162	158–175	168–189	
6	2	156–167	162–180	173–194	198.2
6	3	160–171	167–185	178–199	
6	4	164–175	172–190	182–204	

| Height | | Women | | | |
Feet	Inches	Small Frame	Medium Frame	Large Frame	Actual Average
4	10	92–98	96–107	104–119	
4	11	94–101	98–110	106–122	
5	0	96–104	101–113	109–125	135.2
5	1	99–107	104–116	112–128	
5	2	102–110	107–119	115–131	142.2
5	3	105–113	110–122	118–134	
5	4	108–116	113–126	121–138	149
5	5	111–119	116–130	125–142	
5	6	114–123	120–135	129–146	156
5	7	118–127	124–139	133–150	
5	8	122–131	128–143	137–154	163.2
5	9	126–135	132–147	141–158	
5	10	130–140	136–151	145–163	
5	11	134–144	140–155	149–168	
6	0	138–148	144–159	153–173	

A well-conditioned, muscular athlete and a flabby and out-of-shape person—may well be the same height and weight, or the athlete may even weigh more. Check yourself out in the mirror. If you see signs of flab in places that you wish were lean, you are probably not just vain. Take the "pinch test": pinch the skin and underlying fat in the rear of the upper arm. If you have an inch or more, you have an excess of fat.

How to Lose Weight

The essential controllable factors that determine weight (whether too much or too little) are caloric intake and caloric expenditure. Modifying both daily rates is the best way to approach losing weight. Be leery of fads and gimmicks. There is real danger in crash weight-loss programs. Your body is accustomed to certain foods, even if they are not the best things for it. Abrupt changes can cause serious nutritional deficiencies: sudden alterations of diet can cause biochemical changes equivalent to the intake of powerful drugs.

Diets that call for eating an excessive amount of one type of food or the virtual exclusion of nutrient-bearing foods are bound to create imbalances in your system that will have to be made up for in other ways. This is one reason why people who go on crash diets promptly gain the weight back. Hopping back and forth between weight loss and weight gain—a common occurrence among the chronically obese—puts a tremendous burden on the cardiovascular system.

Most physicians feel that a slow, steady change in eating habits, with careful attention to total calories, fats, and refined sugars, is the best way to reduce weight and maintain a sensible level.

Maintaining acceptable weight should be easy. Nature has equipped us with an elegant mechanism—called an "appestat" by some writers—that regulates our appetites in accordance with the body's needs. Improper eating habits, poor digestion, and excessive stress throw this mechanism out of whack, creating the urge to eat more than you really need. This can also be psychosomatic—most psychologists agree that eating can be an outlet for emotions such as boredom, anxiety, fear, or insecurity.

tips for losing weight

Decide exactly why you want to lose weight; write down why and post copies of it in prominent places. Your reasons for wanting to lose weight must *be important to you.*

Keep a record of what you eat and when. See what triggers improper eating. Substitute other behavior for emotion-based snacking.

Deal with one day at a time. Don't bother thinking about tomorrow; just get through today without slipping.

Be patient. Your body cannot change old habits overnight. If you backslide, don't scold yourself, just persevere.

Set reasonable goals. A pound or two a week is enough—that's 50 to 100 pounds a year!

Adopt a positive attitude. Dieting should not be punishment. It is a means of providing greater health and better appearance.

Get your family and friends to help.

Cut down on fatty foods, and simple sugars and starches.

Eliminate junk foods. They are not only fattening and expensive, but they have virtually no nutritional value, can leave you deficient in vital nutrients, and throw your appetite off kilter.

Weigh yourself weekly and keep a record. Sometimes weight loss is temporarily replaced with fluid in the tissues, so there may be weeks without change. If you keep looking in the mirror for decreased flab, you may not notice the day-to-day progress, but it all adds up.

Do your food shopping after you've eaten. Shop from a prepared list and don't get sidetracked.

Use alcohol sparingly; most drinks are high in caloric content, but you needn't become a teetotaler. In fact, a small intake of alcohol may help reduce the fat content of the blood.

Eat slowly and chew thoroughly. Often we keep eating long past the time we should stop simply because we are going so fast.

Drink lots of water; fruit juice instead of soft drinks.

Reward yourself—use the money saved on junk foods for theater tickets or a new tennis racquet.

Exercise regularly—exercise alone is useless for weight loss, unless done in extraordinary amounts. But it will help tone your muscles, so your newly acquired slim becomes trim.

If you eat lots of junk food, taper off gradually. Nibble on fresh fruit or any acceptable snacks, such as sunflower seeds.

Increase the fiber in your diet. This can prevent intestinal problems and provide enough bulk to alleviate the feeling of emptiness. To add fiber to your diet, eat whole grain cereals and breads instead of white; eat fresh fruits and vegetables (especially cabbage, cauliflower, carrots, apples, figs, and other high-fiber produce); take two or three tablespoons a day of unprocessed bran.

Don't starve yourself. Eat ample amounts of nutritious food. You can't trick your body—if you don't feed it, it will continue to crave the necessary nutrients.

Eat a substantial breakfast. Many executives skip breakfast, or gulp down a donut and coffee because they are in a hurry. By so doing, you keep the blood sugar fluctuating in extremes; if it falls too low, the body is forced to draw from its own reserves for energy, resulting in sugar cravings. Eating a balanced breakfast, with some protein and little or no sugar or starch, will provide energy and keep the blood sugar level even for a longer period. Your cravings for sugary snacks and huge meals will be reduced.

Once you reach your desired weight, establish a regular eating pattern to maintain it and keep you well nourished. Continue to keep track of your weight, and experiment by adding small amounts of previously forbidden foods to see which you can handle and in what amounts.

Eating out is no excuse. Most restaurants have ample amounts of nonfattening fare. Choose your restaurants with discrimination if possible, and when the choice is not yours, order carefully. Your peers will probably respect anyone who takes health seriously; they may even envy your willpower.

where to eat well and keep weight down

Most restaurants can meet a dieter's needs. These cited are favorites with local businessmen watching their waistlines.

Atlanta
    Herren's
    The Midnight Sun
    Clock O Fives, in the Hyatt Regency
Boston
    Top of the Hub, at Prudential Center
    Ritz Carlton
    Locke-Ober's
Chicago
    Kinzie Steak House
    Palmer House Tavern
    Fuji Restaurant
Cleveland
    Cleveland Plaza
    Hollenden House
    Harvey's English
    Oak Room (in Terminal
    Tower, Public Square)
Detroit
    Detroit Hilton
    Sheraton-Cadillac
    Stouffer's
    The Money Tree
Houston
    Warwick Hotel's Vienna and Hunt Rooms
    Houston Oaks Hotel
Los Angeles
    The choice is virtually unlimited in this health-conscious city
New York
    For seafood dieters: Gloucester House at 37 E. 50th
    Sweet's at Fulton and South Streets

Philadelphia
    One of many: Arthur's Steak House
Pittsburgh
    Carlton House Hotel
    Kaufman's Dept. Store (11th floor is a local dieters' favorite)
San Francisco
    Salma Gundi
    Magic Pan
Seattle
    Golden Lion, in the Olympic Hotel
    Jonah and the Whale
    Ivar's Indian Salmon House
Washington, D.C.
    Statler-Hilton (buffet)
    Sheraton Carlton
    Loew's L'Enfant Plaza

protein

Many people fear cutting down on fats and calories because that usually involves cutting down on their main source of protein—meat. The fear is based on a certain amount of truth; protein is usually regarded as the most important nutrient in our diets, and meat is the most common supplier of it. But the average American is in no actual danger of protein deficiency even if he cuts his meat consumption drastically. In fact, it is said that we usually eat entirely too much of it. Nutritionists generally recommend that protein comprise 10 to 15 percent of your daily caloric intake; most Americans eat at least twice that amount.

Proteins are made of chains of nitrogen-containing building blocks called amino acids, as many as 200 of which are strung together to make one protein molecule. Of the 20 known amino acids, the human body can manufacture about twelve from its intake of carbohydrates and nitrogen. The other eight are called "essential" amino acids and must be supplied in complete form in our diets.

When you eat protein, it is broken down into its component amino acids. These are absorbed by the cells, which take them apart and reassemble them into new proteins, as needed. Protein comprises about half the body's dry weight. Each cell contains protein. Without it, new tissues can't be formed to replace worn-out ones. For these and a multitude of other important reasons, protein must be eaten regularly, preferably at each meal, for maximum efficiency. Too much protein, however, can be detrimental. Extra protein, especially from meat sources, will be a source of extra calories, and therefore weight. It will also contribute to extra stores of fat, thus raising the risk of atherosclerosis.

The recommended daily allowance for adults 19 years and over is .36 grams per pound of body weight. To calculate the amount you should consume, simply multiply your weight by .36. In planning a diet to provide that amount, you should try to choose sources that will supply what is needed without unnecessary fats and calories (see box below).

It is generally recommended that one-third of your protein should come from animal sources and the rest from vegetables. Most of us derive 60 to 80 percent from animals. There are many excellent sources of vegetable protein, among them soybeans, nuts, sesame seeds, sunflower seeds, wheat germ, brown rice, and beans such as garbanzos. However, most vegetable proteins are deficient in one or more essential amino acids. For that reason, none of them will suffice by itself. They should be combined in the same meal, or eaten with meat, so that the body can manufacture new protein.

───── fats and calories in protein sources ─────

Type of Food	Fat (grams per oz.)	Protein (grams per oz.)	Calories (per oz.)
Pork	7	7	91
Beef	6	6	78
Lamb	6	6	78
Veal	3	9	63
Organs	1	8	41
Fish (most types)	2	5	38
Crab	0.5	5	25
Lobster	0.5	6	29
Shrimp	0.5	6	31
Chicken or turkey	1	8	41
Canned tuna	3	8	55
Hamburger	6	7	82
Whole milk	1.5	1	21
Skimmed milk	0	1	10
Butter	24	0.2	180
Cottage cheese	0.5	2	12
One egg (boiled)	6	3.5	80
Nuts	18	7	214
Processed American cheese	8.5	6.5	106.5
Plain yogurt (skimmed milk)	0.5	1	14

Rice and beans, corn and beans, whole wheat macaroni with cheese, cereal and milk, yams and beans, or a peanut butter sandwich on whole wheat bread are some examples of non-meat combinations that provide complimentary amino acids (one supplying what the other lacks). Using these protein sources and dairy products at each meal will enable you to cut down on the amount of meat (and fat) you consume without becoming deficient in protein.

low-fat, high-protein casseroles

The following chart, prepared by Anna Gordon, dietician at Columbia Presbyterian Medical Center in New York, will enable you to prepare tasty casseroles with complete proteins derived from non-meat sources. The items in the first two columns supply balanced, complementary protein. Columns three, four, and five provide a variety of ingredients for added flavor and texture. Simply choose one ingredient from each column. Mix together the ingredients from the first four columns, pour into a casserole dish and bake 30 minutes at 375°. Then top with one choice from columns five and bake 15 minutes at 325°. Serves 4–6.

Complementary proteins

1	2	3	4	5
2 cups cooked	1 cup cooked	Sauce: 1 can soup & ¾ c. water	Vegetables to make 1½ c.	3–5 tbsp. topping
Brown Rice	Soybeans	Cream of tomato	Browned celery & green onions	Wheat germ
Macaroni, whole wheat	Lima beans	Cream of potato	Mushrooms & bamboo shoots	Slivered almonds
Corn	Peas	Cream of mushroom	Browned green pepper & garlic	Fresh whole wheat bread crumbs
Spaghetti, whole wheat	Kidney beans	Cream of celery	Cooked green beans	Sesame seeds
Brown rice, converted	Black beans	Cheddar cheese soup	Cooked carrots	Brewers' yeast (debittered)
Noodles, whole wheat	Garbanzos (chick-peas)	Cream of pea	Browned onion & pimiento	Sunflower seeds

─────────────────────────────────── sugar ───

A century ago the average American consumed about five pounds of sugar a year. Today, despite the dramatic rise in sugar prices, the figure is over a hundred pounds a year, a rate of consumption that makes sugar the third major ingredient in the American diet after milk and meat. According to Dr. Emanuel Cheraskin, professor of oral medicine at the University of Alabama, "The American eats more candy than eggs; drinks more soft drinks than milk; downs as much sugar as the combined intake of eggs, all fruits, potatoes, all other vegetables, and whole grain cereals."

Is that bad? Don't we need sugar for energy? Yes, our bodies need sugar to live; we burn sugar to generate the energy necessary for the complex processes within our cells. But we do not need as much as we eat, nor do we need it in the form in which we normally consume it.

"Sugar is an essential nutrient just as is water, but an ocean is too much," writes the popular nutritionist and author Adelle Davis. It is not just a matter of pouring granulated sugar into the things we eat, but of consuming large amounts of refined sugar unknowingly. "A person may consume one or even two cups of sugar daily and still believe they have eaten 'no sugar at all,'" writes Davis. Soft drinks, desserts, cocktails, and virtually all canned and processed foods—soups, vegetables, fruits, crackers—all are made with added sugar. Refined starches— white bread, noodles, spaghetti, rice, pastry—also are hidden sources of sugar, because they turn rapidly into that product once assimilated.

What are the consequences of too much simple sugar? Diabetes, a condition of excess blood sugar, has been considered a possible result, but there is considerable disagreement on the issue. Many experts believe that heredity and obesity, rather than sugar, bring about the diabetic state. Certainly sugar aggravates a diabetes-prone condition.

Hypoglycemia

Interestingly, *low* blood sugar, rather than high, is attracting attention. Dr. Carlton Fredericks, president of the International Academy of Preventive Medicine, estimates that there are at least 20 million Americans who suffer from *hypoglycemia,* or low blood sugar. A study by the U.S. Department of Health, Education and Welfare found that nearly half of 134,000 interviewees had hypoglycemia to one degree or another.

Sugar stimulates the pancreas to secrete insulin, which helps transform the sugar and other substances into usable glucose. Too much sugar causes an overproduction of insulin, which in turn burns up not only the sugar you have just eaten, but some of your reserves of blood sugar as well. The result: too little glucose in the blood. Since glucose is the brain's fuel, significant difficulties can arise during a shortage.

The symptoms of hypoglycemia can be rather severe, according to those who accept it as a legitimate diagnosis (not everyone does). Or they can be mild, but annoying, if the sugar level is only moderately low. Hypoglycemics typically obtain a rush of energy soon after eating, especially if the meal contains sugar or starch. The common "pick-me-up" foods contain sugar for this reason. However, the boost lasts only a short while. The pancreas, overstimulated by the influx of sugar, secretes excessive amounts of insulin. Too much sugar is drawn from the blood, and fatigue, tension, irritability, disorientation, and other symptoms follow.

When this sequence occurs repeatedly, permanent low blood sugar, or hypoglycemia, can result. In severe cases, the symptoms can include vertigo, headaches, cramps, tremors, blurred vision, and cold sweats. In most cases, psychological symptoms like lethargy, foggy thinking, depression, confusion, and anxiety are associated with low blood sugar. Some have fainted or have had their hearts start pounding so heavily they feared they were having a heart attack. In most cases, fluctuations of mood and energy level—often from one extreme to the other—are the rule.

Blood sugar and stress have a feedback effect on one another. When the brain fails to obtain sufficient glucose, the body goes into an emergency state that stimulates the adrenals as in the classic fight-or-flight response. That is why hypoglycemics often become hyperactive. The result is weakened adrenals, and a consequent inefficiency in responding to stress. Excessive stress can so weaken the endocrine system that the hormones necessary for converting body starch into sugar are not sufficiently produced. Hence blood sugar remains low.

Thus, according to many authorities, people under a great deal of stress and who consume large amounts of simple sugars, starch, alcohol, and coffee are likely to have low blood sugar. If you have a persistent sweet tooth, if your energy level fluctuates, if fatigue is a consistent problem, if you become irritable and disoriented when you delay eating, if you feel better after a meal only to suffer a slump soon afterward, or if you become depressed and lethargic unexpectedly you may want to have your doctor administer a glucose-tolerance test to check out your blood sugar.

Blood Sugar Controversy

The concept of hypoglycemia is not universally accepted among physicians. Many consider it too simplistic a diagnosis, others feel that it is not only valid, but a problem of epidemic proportions, frequently overlooked because physicians are not trained to notice nutritional causes. They claim that many hypoglycemics go from doctor to doctor, or from psychiatrist to psychiatrist, only to be told there is nothing wrong with them but "nervous tension" or "overwork."

Those with hypoglycemia are told to adopt a strict diet: absolutely no sugar; no caffeine; drastically reduced starches; limited amounts of dried fruits; a lot of protein, which metabolizes slowly and will not induce radical shifts of insulin; and snacks of milk, juice, cheese, or nuts at regular intervals to keep the blood sugar at an even level throughout the day.

Even if you do not check out with low blood sugar on a lab test, cutting down or eliminating sugar will probably do you a lot of good anyway. The McGovern report recommends reducing sugar consumption by about 40 percent.

Experts agree that our blood sugar needs are best met by obtaining it from the complex carbohydrates found in vegetables, whole grain breads, beans, bananas, and other produce. A well-balanced diet should supply ample amounts; we don't need all that much sugar. It has only one purpose, says Ms. Davis—"to be used to produce energy when a supply of energy is demanded. Otherwise it may be stored as fat for the duration of your life. It cannot build body tissue or improve general health and attractiveness."

Sugar and Disease

Perhaps the best reason to cut down on your sugar intake is that it has been implicated in heart disease. John Yudkin, professor of biochemistry at the University of London, found in 1959 that people who consume 120 pounds of sugar a year have six times the chance of coming down with coronary heart disease as people who use 60 pounds. Those who ingest 150 pounds or more have a 15 times greater chance. Sugar apparently raises the fat level of the blood and increases the amount of cholesterol-containing lipoproteins.

Drs. Friedman and Rosenman have noted that their Type A patients are particularly prone to this mechanism. "There is considerable evidence suggesting that the excess ingestion of various types of simple sugars is particularly apt to elevate the serum cholesterol of Type A subjects." They advise anyone with Type A tendencies, or with any indication of being coronary prone, to avoid all but small quantities of sugar and other simple carbohydrates.

Sugar has also been implicated in deficiencies of key vitamins and minerals, notably thiamine and niacine. The final word on sugar belongs to Nobel Prize winning biologist Linus Pauling:

> I believe that if people were to avoid sucrose—hardly ever spoon out a spoonful of sugar from the sugar bowl onto anything, avoid sweet des-

serts except when you're a guest somewhere, avoid buying foods that say 'sugar' as one of the contents—they could cut down on the incidence of disease and increase life expectancy.

salt

The highest incidence of hypertension in the world occurs in Northern Japan where the salt intake is among the world's highest. Salt is often cited as a cause of hypertension, although some feel that it becomes a factor only when taken in large amounts by those already disposed toward high blood pressure.

Most of us pour entirely too much salt on our foods, and when we don't it is done for us in prepared foods. We don't need it for anything other than taste. Writes nutritionist Dr. Mary S. Rose, "The amount of sodium chloride taken in the form of common salt is far in excess of human requirements for sodium and chloride." You can get plenty of sodium from foods containing natural mineral salts—uncooked fruits and vegetables, nuts, and seeds.

Foods containing a lot of sodium should be avoided by anyone with a tendency toward high blood pressure. In addition to table salt beware of catsups, cold meats, canned soups, salted nuts, and dishes containing baking soda. Potassium-chloride salt substitutes are available. The McGovern report recommends that everyone reduce salt intake by 50 to 85 percent, to about three grams per day.

Most people who are placed on low salt diets report that their food tastes bland at first. That apparently lasts only a week or two, after which the taste buds adjust and the natural unsalted taste of food is enjoyed.

vitamins and minerals

Among those who have studied nutrition, it is widely accepted that stress can create an extra demand for certain vitamins and minerals that are needed for normal functioning. Under such demand, the body will call upon its stores of those chemicals, thus running the risk of depleting its supplies. Furthermore, certain vitamins and minerals are needed to maintain the proper functioning of the organs and glands that are instrumental in managing stress.

Vitamins are organic food substances that are essential for proper growth and maintenance of health. They are not foods in the sense that fats, proteins, or carbohydrates are foods; they are built into the structure of cells where they help certain essential processes take place. We obtain these substances (15 vitamins have been recognized, while an unknown amount remain undiscovered) by eating plants, which manufacture their own vitamins, or by eating animals, which have obtained theirs from eating plants.

No one disputes the need for vitamins. What is disputed, however, and rather hotly, is whether or not we need to supplement our ordinary diets with vitamin pills. On one side are those who feel that no one needs supplements as long as he eats a "balanced diet." Says Robert B. Bradfield, professor of nutrition at the U. of C. at Berkeley:

> If you eat a mixed diet of fruits, vegetables, and protein sources, the odds are very high that you don't need supplemental vitamins. If you feel you don't eat a mixed diet, the typical multivitamin tablet, sold widely and based on government-recommended allowances, is sufficient.

On the other side is megavitamin therapy, wherein huge doses of vitamins and minerals—often many times the recommended daily allowance—are used to correct imbalances and deficiencies that are said to cause or contribute to illness. These therapies, championed by the school of orthomolecular psychiatry, claim great success in treating everything from schizophrenia to the common cold. Detractors point out that few of those claims have been scientifically verified (to which the proponents respond: no one in the medical establishment or the powerful drug companies will sponsor the needed research), and that the overzealous dispensing of supplements might be as biochemically hazardous as the indiscriminate use of drugs, which the vitamin therapists deplore.

Theoretically, no one would deny that our diets *should* supply all the vitamins and minerals we need. Obviously, nature did not intend for us to manufacture tablets in order to be healthy. But, say the advocates of supplements, nature did not intend for us to undergo severe stress. Further, they argue, our diets are far from ideal; they do not supply the vitamins we need.

"If wholesome foods were available, supplements would rarely be needed," wrote Adelle Davis, lamenting the fact that they appear to be necessary. "As I see it," she added, "thousands of adults and millions of children in our country have never once had a mouthful of genuinely wholesome food. Everything we eat is tinkered with in one way or another. With every tinkering come losses."

Nutritionists cite the use of insecticides, packaging and shipping procedures, additives, and other regular features of mass food production as vitamin depleters. As a result of improper eating habits (like too much sugar) and stress, the theory goes, our systems become like faulty motors that get poor mileage from even the best gasoline. "It's not so much what you eat," says Samuel Bursuk, consulting nutritionist to the North Nassau Mental Health Center on Long Island, "It's what you *assimilate.* Most people have what we call 'malabsorption syndrome.' They eat like pigs and they don't get the benefits of the food."

Certain vitamins and minerals are said to be vital to the body's antistress mechanism. Be sure your diet contains ample quantities of each, and take supplements if you have doubts.

stress-related vitamins and minerals

Stress-related Vitamins and Minerals	U.S. Recommended Daily Allowance	Food Sources	Why Needed
A	Adult males: 5000 international units (IU) Adult females: 5000 IUs	green and yellow veg.; eggs; fish liver oils; organ meats (i.e. liver)	Said to be of therapeutic and preventive value in stress-induced disease, infectious disease, respiratory infections. Studies have shown that large doses helped reduce thymus shrinkage, a consequence of severe stress, in rats.
B_1* (thiamine)	Adult males: 1.4 mg. Adult females: 1.0 mg.	whole grains, liver, beans, brewer's yeast, wheat germ, green vegetables.	Associated with emotional stability, nervous disorders, alcoholism, fatigue, abnormal heart beat, depression, forgetfulness, confusion (the brain is fed by glucose, which can't be converted into energy without B_1).
B_3 (niacin)	Adult males: 18 mg. Adult females: 13 mg.	yeast, organ meats, fish, nuts, wheat germ, soybeans.	Deficiencies are associated with personality changes, apprehension, moods, confusion, worry, forgetfulness, depression. Has been useful in treating insomnia, schizophrenia, other stress disorders. Said to be useful in overcoming excessive alcohol consumption.

*All the B vitamins are closely associated with stress; yeast, liver, soy flour, and kidney are best sources of B complex. If taking supplement, be sure to take one that supplies *all* B vitamins. They work together synergistically.

stress-related vitamins and minerals (continued)

B6 (pyridoxine)	Adult males: 2 mg. Adult females: 2 mg.	organ meats, whole grains, walnuts, peanuts, wheat germ, bananas, fish, sunflower seeds.	Aids in metabolism of fat and carbohydrates; important to brain functions. Deficiencies associated diabetes, anemia, nervous disorders depression, insomnia, nausea, dizziness, asthma. Said to be one of the most prevalent deficiencies in U.S. Prevents ulcers in rats.
B12	Adult males: 5 mg. Adult females: 5 mg.	yeast, liver, wheat germ, milk, eggs.	Important for nervous system. Deficiencies associated with anemia, nervous disorders, mental illness, neuritis. It is said to be needed for proper functioning of the immune system.
Pantothnic acid	Adult males: 10 mg. Adult females: 10 mg.	liver, kidney, brewer's yeast, sunflower seeds, peanuts.	Necessary for proper functioning of all cells. Neither fat nor sugar can be converted into energy without it. Called the "antistress vitamin" because of importance to adrenal glands and immune system. Absence makes one more vulnerable to stress because adrenals don't function properly.
C	Adult males: 60 mg. Adult females: 55 mg.	citrus fruit, rose hips, green pepper, broccoli, spinach, tomato.	Important in fighting infection, repairing tissue, maintaining healthy adrenal glands. Stress known to destroy body's reserves, increasing vulnerability. Deficiencies thought to be associated with cholesterol buildup, and atherosclerosis.

E	Adult males: 30 IUs Adult females: 25 IUs	green leafy veg., whole grains (rice, wheat, etc.), wheat germ, safflower oil, peanuts.	Deficiencies associated with anemia, liver and kidney damage, muscle degeneration. Said to be an anticlotting agent. Dr. Richard Passwater studied 17,894 subjects and found rate of heart disease proportionate to amount of time taking vitamin E. May improve blood flow and oxygen utilization.
Calcium	Adults: 1800 mg.	milk, cheese, all dairy products, bone meal, eggs, figs, almonds, soybeans, cauliflower, broccoli.	A natural sedative. Important for nervous system. Deficiencies associated with nervousness, fatigue, grouchiness, tension. Said to be important in regulating the heartbeat. Important for sound sleep. (Absorption of calcium requires sufficient vitamin D and magnesium).
Potassium	Adults: 5000 mg.	green leafy veg., fish, nuts, fruits, unrefined grains, meat.	Deficiencies associated with fatigue, listlessness, insomnia, low blood sugar. Said to be essential for health of heart muscles.
Magnesium	Adult males: 350 mg. Adult females: 300 mg.	fruits and veg.(esp. spinach), dates, prunes, kelp, seeds.	Called "nature's tranquilizer". Deficiencies associated with irritability, hyperexcitability, apprehension, belligerence, tremors, insomnia, irregular pulse, emotional disorders. Said by some to be associated with heart attack. Needed for absorption of calcium and potassium.

A Word on Supplements

The data on the therapeutic uses of vitamins and the connections between deficiencies and disease are hotly debated. The information in the table above was derived from sources *partial* to nutritional therapy. It is only fair to mention that those views have staunch opponents in the medical establishment, and an even greater number of cold skeptics. Moderation should be used in taking supplements. According to a *Newsweek* report (December 14, 1977), too much vitamin A has been known to cause fatal liver damage; excessive vitamin D intake can raise blood calcium levels enough to cause cardiac arrest; astronomical doses of vitamin C—imbibed by many to combat colds—is alleged to block the action of vitamin B_{12}.

Another point to keep in mind is that taking extra vitamins may correct deficiencies, but there is an upper limit beyond which the vitamin is, if not destructive, at least useless. Chances are, if you (1) eat an adequately nutritious diet; (2) stay away from vitamin depleters like alcohol, sugar, and simple starches; and (3) lead a healthy life-style, you will be getting sufficient vitamins and minerals. Nonetheless, a good multivitamin is excellent insurance, especially for executives who are exposed to a good deal of stress, and who are often forced to eat on the run or not at all.

Supplement the multivitamin with C and B-complex, the two that seem to be most closely related to stress. Your C should be derived from rose hips if possible. Remember that the B vitamins work together; each is relatively useless unless the others are present in sufficient quantity. Some of the cheaper brands of B-complex are out of balance. Brewer's yeast is the best source.

Many experts claim that natural vitamins, made from organic sources, are preferable to synthetic ones. Others dispute the claim. "In general," concludes Adelle Davis, "it seems wise to use natural sources when you can, but be willing to use synthetic ones whenever you need to."

If you are interested in consulting with a doctor who is nutrition oriented, contact the Huxley Institute for Biosocial Research, 1114 First Avenue, New York, N.Y. 10021; or the Academy for Orthomolecular Psychiatry, North Nassau Mental Health Center, 1691 Northern Blvd., Manhasset, N.Y. 11030.

summary: intelligent eating

"The well-balanced executive is never distracted by hunger during working hours," writes Dr. Robert Collier Page. "Neither is he drowsy and dull from overeating. He sticks to a happy medium between undernourishment and satiety. How this is accomplished varies from individual to individual."

There is no diet suitable for every individual; your tastes, habits, and needs are your own, and any intelligent nutritional program must take those into account. However, that realization has given many people a good excuse for indulging in tasty, but destructive, eating. "I eat what my body tells me it needs," says the cavalier eater. "If it tells me to eat ice cream, it must need it." Not necessarily. It could be that your body is out of balance and its cravings do not reflect its true needs. And yet, somehow, you must strike a balance between nutrition and enjoyment; a healthy meal eaten grudgingly will probably sour in the belly.

---

tips on how and when to eat

Be moderate. It is better to eat smaller meals more frequently than to stuff yourself at any one sitting. The latter places excessive demands on the digestive system and throws the blood sugar off balance.

Eat when you are hungry, if possible, not just when the clock tells you to.

If you anticipate a stressful event coming up, eat a little more than you ordinarily would; if you anticipate a lull, eat a little less. This may run counter to your appetite at those times, but is a precaution against skipping meals before stress, and overeating out of boredom.

During nonstrenuous or extra-sedentary periods, cut down on fats and starches. They will build up and create a useless store of calories. Counteract lulls with exercise. If you do not use your body regularly, digestion will be sluggish.

Chew thoroughly and eat slowly. Digestion begins in the mouth.

If possible, break for 10–15 minutes before lunch and dinner. Relax. Mealtime should be calm and gracious. If you are under strain the flow of digestive juices will be impeded and many enzymes will not be produced. "Fecal analysis of a group of successful businessmen revealed quantities of undigested meat fibers," reports Adelle Davis. "Such factors as worry, fatigue, and perhaps the stress of competition combined to prevent their (expensive) steaks from digesting."

Favor fresh foods over packaged or processed foods. Fruits and vegetables are just as easy to prepare as canned or frozen ones and the gains in taste and nutrition make the extra time spent shopping for them well worthwhile.

Read labels carefully. Chemical additives are highly questionable, and a great deal of unsuspected sugar and salt is imbibed in canned packaged items.

Eat with gusto and enjoy!

—— **recommended reading: chapter seven** ——

Diet for a Small Planet, Frances Moore Lappé (New York: Ballantine Books, 1971).

Let's Eat Right to Keep Fit, Adelle Davis (New York: Harcourt Brace Jovanovich, 1954).

Live Longer Now, Leonard, Hofer, and Pritikin (New York: Grosset & Dunlap, 1977).

Orthomolecular Psychiatry, Linus Pauling (available from the Huxley Institute, 1114 First Ave., New York, N.Y. 10021).

Psychodietetics: Food as the Key to Emotional Health, Cheraskin, Ringsdorf, and Brecher (New York: Stein & Day, 1974).

Sugar Blues, William Dufty (New York: Warner, 1976).

Supernutrition: Megavitamin Revolution, Richard Passwater (New York: Dial, 1975).

The Complete Book of Vitamins, Prevention Magazine (Emmaus, Pa.: Rodale Press, 1977).

mental relaxation techniques

self-evaluation: are you relaxed?

1. Do you hesitate to take time out to do nothing?
2. Do you find it difficult to relax?
3. Do you feel guilty when you take time out to relax?
4. Do your hands or feet get cold even in a warm room?
5. Are your palms or brow chronically moist?
6. Are there deeply etched wrinkle lines on your forehead? Around your eyes or mouth?
7. In the course of the average day, do you often experience tightening of the stomach muscles?
     Rapid heartbeat?
     Shortness of breath?
     Trembling hands and fingers?
     Restless legs?
     Other signs of tension?
8. Do your neck and shoulder muscles get tight frequently?
     Do you feel the urge to stretch or massage them?
9. Do you clench your jaw or grind your teeth habitually?
10. During a lull in your workday, can you easily turn off the pressure and just let go?
11. Do you practice any formal method of relaxation?
12. Have you ever looked into Transcendental Meditation or other relaxation techniques?
     Do such practices have a negative connotation to you?
13. Are your muscles—particularly arms and legs—chronically tensed?
     When at your desk, or waiting for a train, notice if your arms and legs are braced, as though poised for action. Bracing is usually unconscious, yet it can drain energy and lead to chronic tension. Some time when you think you are relaxed, close your eyes and let your attention

scan your body slowly. Become aware of each part of your body, and notice the sensations in all the muscles. Where is there unnecessary tension or tautness? This will help you become aware of the areas in which tension manifests in your body.

the ability to relax

Psychologist Carl Thoreson, currently working on a federally funded experiment exploring the relationship between behavior and heart disease, feels that the first step toward prevention of stress disorders is to take the time to relax. His belief is echoed throughout the medical community. Yet it has been pointed out over and over again that the people who most need to relax, notably hard-working executives, are the first ones to resist it.

The executive is likely to complain, "If I had the time to relax, I wouldn't be tense in the first place." Thoreson believes that much of that time urgency is a self-inflicted Type A trait, usually blown out of proportion to reality. He suggests that you realize you are the type of person who is inclined to say, "I am too busy to relax," and ask yourself candidly whether it wouldn't be cost-effective to take 15–20 minutes out to refresh your mind and body.

In the long run, you save time by relaxing. When weighed down by problems, you are not necessarily clear-minded enough to come up with the best solutions. A good break at the right time can be more effective than forcing yourself to plod through when your brain is overloaded. Some of the greatest scientific discoveries and works of art dawned on the creators when work was the farthest thing from their minds. The structure of the DNA molecule, for example, came to its discoverer when he lay abed cutting out paper dolls to get his mind off his insoluble problem. The dolls dangled from his hand in the shape of a helix. Instant revelation! The DNA molecule is helix shaped.

Perhaps that is why management consultant Christopher Hegerty feels that "the single most important ingredient necessary to be a successful executive is the ability to operate on an ever-deepening level of personal calmness." For decades, doctors and psychologists were accustomed to telling people to "learn how to relax," but they could not tell them how. It is, as most readers undoubtedly know, not a simple thing for an overly tense executive to turn it off. The emergence of systematic, teachable techniques is an important breakthrough in health management. As with other discoveries, the realization that human beings are capable of relaxing through volition has spurred a wide variety of techniques and programs, ranging from the tried and true to dubious imitations that border on charlatanism.

It will be some time before scientists know all there is to know about the effects of these techniques, or about their relationship to one another. For now, it is safe to say that proven methods are available to elicit, in essence, the reverse of the stress, or fight-or-flight, response. Learning to use them is a significant aid in reducing wear and tear.

abdominal breathing

The conception of life is so closely bound up with that of respiration that the very word "expiration" has come to connote the extinction of life, and "inspiration" its elevation to a super-human level. Respiration is a process common to all forms of life, the reason for which is that the chemical basis of life is essentially an oxidation of tissue.——*Encyclopedia Britannica*

Most individuals, particularly when under stress, tend to breathe in short, shallow breaths. They breathe primarily by expanding their chests. This thoracic breathing, as it is called, prevents the lungs from filling up completely. Stale, used air remains unexpelled, and oxidation of tissues is incomplete. Muscle tension is one result of this improper breathing. In reverse, learning to breathe completely is useful for reducing tension. It is also good for the brain. Though it weighs only a few pounds, the brain uses about 20 percent of the oxygen we take in.

Take five or ten minutes once or twice a day to practice the abdominal breathing method below until it becomes habitual. Just before lunch and sometime in the late afternoon when you begin to slump are good times. It is best to practice seated upright. Once this breathing becomes routine, it can be used to reverse the stress response whenever it is triggered.

---

abdominal breathing

For practice purposes, place your hands on your abdomen, right below the navel. The fingertips of each hand should touch one another.

Breathe through your nose; many people habitually breathe through their mouths, an almost sure sign of stress overload, and not nearly as healthy.

Inhale very slowly; as you do, push the abdomen out as though it were a balloon expanding. Your fingers should separate.

As the abdomen expands, your diaphragm will move downward, allowing fresh air to enter the bottom part of the lungs. Keeping your back straight will aid the process of maximizing inhalation.

As the breath continues, expand the chest. More air should now enter, filling the middle part of the lungs.

Slightly contracting the abdomen, raise your shoulders and collar-bones. This should fill the upper part of the lungs.

At this point, the entire respiratory mechanism has been employed and no portion of the lungs is left unfilled. Hold the breath for about five seconds.

Exhalation is as important as inhalation. Proper exhalation not only expels all used air, it opens space for fresh new air to enter. After holding the breath, begin slowly to exhale through the nose. As you do so, draw in the abdomen. This will lift the diaphragm. The expanded rib cage will return to its normal position, and the lungs will empty.

Remember to exhale slowly, and let all the air empty out. If comfortable, hold it a second or two before beginning the inhalation again. When you resume, remember to inhale slowly and completely.

Your first few practice sessions may leave you with a slight dizzy feeling. That is normal. Don't strain to retain the breath or to go any slower than is comfortable.

After some practice, abdominal breathing will become automatic. It can be used when you are under stress, or immediately preceding a stressful event, without breaking your routine. Indeed, a few complete breaths are calming and go unnoticed in the midst of a committee meeting or a phone call. Psychologists who conduct stress programs for major corporations have reported that the procedure has produced excellent results.

self-massage

Here is a full body massage that is simple enough to do in your chair or sofa to relieve muscular tension. In doing this, be sure not to apply too much pressure. Many people erroneously believe that massage is good only if it hurts. While leaning into a particularly tense muscle can work wonders, be sure you don't press too hard on tendons, ligaments, or bones. Women should be particularly gentle around the breasts, and everyone should avoid pressure at the lymph glands (under the jaw and the armpits in particular). On the large muscles, such as the thighs, considerable pressure may be applied. But do it gradually or else the muscle will tense up.

self-massage

Start at the top of the head. With both hands, press firmly with your palms and fingertips, moving in a slow circular motion. Move the hands forward, continuing to press, over the forehead and face. Continue over the neck and chest, stopping at the heart. Don't hesitate to linger any place that feels particularly in need of massage.

Return your hands to the top of your head. This time move down the back of the head, pressing as you go. Give lots of time and pressure to the neck and shoulder area. Those who lean over a desk a good portion of their days accumulate considerable tension there. Using your fingertips, press deeply in rotating motion on the trapezius muscles that run from the base of the neck to the edge of the shoulder. Cross your hands over if it is easier—your right hand massaging your left shoulder and vice versa.

Grasp the fingertips of your left hand with your right hand. Move up the back of the left hand and on up the arm, with your thumb on the underside and your fingers on the top. Move slowly up to the shoulder, pausing again at the trapezius if you still feel stiff in that area. Then come down the left side of the chest, pressing with the fingertips as you go, and end at the heart. Now repeat the process with the fingers of your right hand beneath the left arm and the thumb on top. Then switch hands, massaging the right both above and below.

Place your hands on your abdomen, with your fingertips touching below the navel. Massage your belly gently and move up to the chest.

Place your hands on your lower back, joining fingertips at the coccyx. Massage the lower back deeply with your fingertips. This is another area that gets sore from sedentary work. Then move up the back, massaging as you go, until you can reach no further.

Grasp the toes of your left foot with hour hands, placing the left hand on top and the right underneath. Give your feet a good tough massage. Tight shoes, failure to walk as often as you should, and poor circulation produce cramps and tension in the feet. Reportedly, there are nerve endings in the feet connected to all parts of the body. Some physiologists believe that working out the tension around those nerve endings can improve circulation to the specific organs associated with them. Press deeply, perhaps even using your knuckles. Avoid the bones and ligaments, but press deeply into other areas even if it hurts somewhat.

Now begin moving up the leg, over the ankles and calf, massaging as you go. Continue over the knee and up the thigh. Circulation in the leg, which gets sluggish if you fail to use the muscles for long periods of time, is stimulated by this.

Switch to the right foot, placing the right hand on top and the left underneath. Repeat the foot and leg massage.

This all-over massage can be done any time. Some apply it at bedtime, perhaps immediately following a warm bath, to encourage restful sleep. If you and your spouse wish to learn how to administer massage to one another, the book to get is *The Massage Book,* by George Downing (Random House).

progressive relaxation

You may have noticed that your muscles maintain a certain degree of rigidity even when you are in a state of rest. If you haven't, look for it the next time you think you are relaxed. In all likelihood, you will observe unnecessary tautness, particularly in the arms and legs. Your muscles will still display a certain resistance to being moved, whereas in complete relaxation there is no resistance.

Edmund Jacobson noticed this as a student at Harvard in 1908. In his long career as a physiologist-physician, Dr. Jacobson developed a systematic program for retraining muscles to obtain complete relaxation. He was able to measure the amount of electrical activity in a muscle and detect what he called "residual tension," the tension that a person is unaware of, even in a state of apparent relaxation.

In *Progressive Relaxation* (University of Chicago Press, 1929), Jacobson wrote:

> The purpose of relaxation is to do away with certain activities that place an undue tax upon the organism. Since relaxation is the intensive form of rest, we may assume that it will be indicated as a rule where rest is indicated. . . . It is well for the physician to bear in mind that patients who are obviously restless and emotional are not the only ones who are in need of intensive rest.

He recommended using progressive relaxation to supplement medical treatment for a wide range of disorders including anxiety, hypertension, insomnia, colitis, and headaches. The success was such that his techniques have been widely used and imitated ever since.

The key to PR is recognizing even the most fugitive signs of residual tension. By so doing, you can eliminate progressively deeper levels of tension with little or no effort. As with modern biofeedback, the key is the mental recognition of subtle physiological changes.

---

progressive relaxation

Here is a basic progressive relaxation exercise. Set aside practice sessions of 45 minutes if possible (but preferably not just after a meal —or you may just fall asleep). Arrange not to be disturbed.

Loosen your clothing and lie down on a comfortable bed or sofa. Do not fold your arms or cross your legs. Keep your arms at your sides, palms down, a few inches from the body.

Relax. Let your weight sink into the bed. Be sure not to exert any effort in trying to relax; don't admonish yourself, or try to hurry the process along in any way. Just be loose.

After a few minutes, slowly stiffen the muscles in both arms. Don't move your arms, and don't clench your fists.

Hold at a very slight degree of stiffness for about ten seconds. Stiffen a little more, and again hold for ten seconds (don't overdo it).

Observe how your arms feel during that ten seconds. You will probably notice a dull, taut sensation. Some have described it as mild soreness or tenderness. Consciously recognizing these signs of contracted muscles and active nerves is the first step in learning deep relaxation.

Now allow your arms to relax gradually. Notice that the sensations of stiffness begin to become less intense. Rest in the relaxed state for one or two minutes.

Repeat the entire procedure; tighten and hold in progressive stages, hold the third for half a minute, and then relax gradually.

Repeat a third time. During the relaxation stage following the stiffening procedure, continue to let your arms relax, past the point that you ordinarily call relaxation.

As you continue to practice this exercise, you will recognize increasingly deeper levels of tension—the taut, dull feeling will be observable even when it exists only in traces. Similarly, the feeling of relaxation will become more clear. You will be able to distinguish between completely relaxed states and those in which residual tension remains. Without effort, simply by intention and "letting go," you will notice that as you acquire competence the residual tension will also diminish.

Once you feel you have mastered the arms, go on to other muscle groups. The legs, abdomen, chest, and facial muscles should each be tensed and relaxed in the same progressive manner.

After a while you should be able to discontinue the period of tensing that precedes the relaxation. This tensing serves only to acquaint you with what tension feels like. With practice, you will be able to relax every muscle group completely, without effort.

Here is a way to apply the procedure to the facial muscles:

Pull up your eyebrows, wrinkling the forehead. Hold for a minute. Notice the feeling of tension in the forehead muscles.

Gradually let the forehead relax. Remain in the relaxed state for a few minutes.

Close your eyelids very tightly. Hold for thirty seconds. Observe the tension in the muscles.

Relax, but keep the eyes closed lightly. Hold for a few minutes.

Repeat these procedures until you feel all the residual tension is gone.

> *As before, you should eventually eliminate the initial tensing period.*

Remember never to exert effort in relaxing. If some of your muscles seem particularly stubborn and prone to tightening up, it is indicative of deep-seated tension. It might take time to remove such deep residual tension. But *trying* will only *add* to the tension; the effort will cause the muscles to respond as though in an emergency state.

biofeedback

Not long after scientists developed sophisticated machinery with which to measure minute changes in the body's internal activities, researchers like Dr. Neal Miller and Dr. Barbara Brown of UCLA Medical School realized that such technology had applications beyond diagnosis of illness and the advancement of our knowledge of physiology. It could be used by individuals as a way to learn, *and control,* bodily functions that had once been considered involuntary. The clinical application of these discoveries has come to be known as biofeedback.

It has had a tremendous impact on the medical and psychiatric communities, with burgeoning experimentation and an ever expanding range of application. And it has found its way into the business world. Many companies use biofeedback equipment to train employees to regulate muscle tension or blood pressure. Executives at the Chicago headquarters of McDonalds Hamburger, Inc., for example, take relaxation breaks, hooked up to machines. A *New York Times* writer predicted a time when "corporations, law firms and television studios will have a cot and an EMG (muscle tension machine) to permit quick naps and preventative medication for harassed workers during the day."

The responses to biofeedback developments range from jubilation to cynicism. Proponents see it as a sort of technological panacea that could eventually enable us to mentally regulate everything from cancer to warts. The opponents are alarmed at technology's invasion of our very minds, and the specter of perilous misuse of such equipment. Most scientists are somewhere between these extremes. To Dr. Barbara Brown, one of the giant names in biofeedback research, the implications of what has been discovered are astounding; they open up vast new dimensions in self-treatment and communication of mind and body. Of the current reliance on machinery, she feels, "It is merely a temporary technologic station along the path toward knowledge of the inner being."

What Is Biofeedback?

It is actually the application to human beings of principals long known to biologists and engineers. "The expression developed in the field of engineering," writes Dr. Brown, "to define control systems that operate via feedback mechanisms.... The most common example is the thermostat."

In a sense, biofeedback is merely an extension of processes familiar to all of us. We know, for example, when we are having trouble breathing by signs conveyed from our respiratory system; we know how fast our heartbeat is if we put our hand to our chest; we can feel our temperature rise; or when our stomach is full. We take this information and act upon it, often with direct intervention, such as taking a deep breath or eating. But we can't see, taste, feel, hear, or smell our brain waves, or the subtle activity of muscle cells, or our blood pressure. With the use of biofeedback equipment, previously undetectable events can be perceived.

Dr. Sidney Lecker, who uses biofeedback at the StressControl Center in New York, calls it "an electronic window through which we can observe internal bodily processes." Dr. Neal Miller, a pioneer in biofeedback research, compared it to learning to putt. "If both the golfer and coach are blindfolded," writes Dr. Miller, "they will not know whether any putt succeeds or fails. Such knowledge of results, or feedback, serves as a reward or punishment and is necessary if the golfer is to learn."

Biofeedback equipment can monitor events such as brain waves, heartbeat, muscular tension, or skin temperature. These events are then transformed into readily observable signals—lights, tones, wavy lines on a monitor. Once you can "see" your brain waves, or "hear" your blood pressure, you can presumably control these processes, because you can tell if you are succeeding or failing. Eventually, say the biofeedback advocates, you can easily control many such processes, *even without the equipment.*

The electromyograph (EMG) is the most widely used of the biofeedback machines. Apparently, the discrimination of muscular tension is the easiest and quickest to learn; once mastered, other types of training are often introduced. According to Dr. Rosalind Forbes, "As general tension is more easily handled through the use of biofeedback devices, individuals are able to retrain all these sections of the nervous system—striate, autonomic, and central."

Biofeedback procedures have been found helpful in treating cardiac arrhythmias. The patient is fed back information in the form of red, green, and yellow lights, indicating when the heart rate is too fast, too slow, or normal. The idea is simply to keep the yellow light on as much as possible. How does the patient learn how to keep the light on? Through the same basic steps involved in all biofeedback training. In the words of Barbara Brown:

commonly used forms of biofeedback

Name	Method	Function
Galvanic Skin Response (GSR) (Also known as electrodermal response system)	Measures skin resistance to electric current by use of electrodes attached to fingertips.	Skin resistance is a function of moisture of skin, which is considered an indication of nervousness (hence its use as a lie detection device). Rise in skin resistance is signalled by a rise in feedback tone. Used in stress reduction, relaxation training.
Skin temperature (called electro-thermal)	Detects changes in peripheral skin temperature with a thermistor on the finger.	Fingertip temperature is associated with activity of the smooth muscles in the peripheral arteries. Arteries contract under stress, dilate with relaxation. Used to reduce tension and to eliminate migraine headaches.
Electroencephalograph (EEG)	Detects electrical activity on brain's cortex with electrodes attached to scalp. Indicated in form of brain wave patterns.	Certain brain wave patterns are associated with states of mind such as relaxation, creativity, etc. Most commonly sought in training is alpha state.
Electromyograph (EMG)	Measures muscle tension, in form of electrical impulses generated by muscle. Electrodes on forearm or forehead fed back lights, tones, clicks, etc.	Individual learns to reduce muscle tension through feedback. Sometimes relaxation techniques are taught in conjunction with biofeedback training. Used for relaxation.

If you continue to work with the device, as, for example, 15 or 30 minutes a day, then over time some association appears to develop between certain changes in the body sign and different subjective feelings, either consciously or subconsciously recognized.... In time you develop control over fluctuations of the sign, and often may learn to exercise precise control, at will, over how the body sign changes.

Perhaps the best results have come with migraine headaches. Two methods have been used—direct relaxation of the forehead muscles, and hand warming. Apparently, the latter produces a generalized change in the degree of dilation of blood vessels, thus relieving the cause of migraines.

Other disorders known to respond well to biofeedback are hypertension, nerve damage, partial paralysis, gastrointestinal difficulties, and tension headaches. However, many feel the technique may have more far-ranging applications, in, for example, disorders of the musculature, respiratory, and cardiovascular systems. Says a hopeful Dr. Brown: "The learned control over blood pressure, heart rate, and peripheral vasodilation and vasoconstriction will add immeasureably to a [cardiovascular] patient's comfort and life expectancy."

In essence, biofeedback is seen as a major step in self-care and drugless therapy. A person so well tuned to physical changes will, presumably, be able to detect the early warning signs of illness and eliminate them by conscious volition. It is being used more and more by normal, healthy people as a way to train themselves to respond to stress appropriately. They are, in a sense, resetting their thermostats—setting their response mechanism to stress at a higher level.

Is Biofeedback Dangerous?

Like most medical innovations, biofeedback is approached with caution even by those who are using it. Says Dr. Peter Hauri:

> Therapeutic claims often overstate beyond belief small kernels of sound, scientific evidence found in laboratories and clinical research. Clinicians will do well to keep a keen, but very critical, eye on future developments, guarding both against excessive gullibility as well as against wholesale rejection of the field (where excellent scientific work currently mingles with obvious quackery).

Biofeedback instruments are all totally passive: no electrical energy passes from the instrument to the body. There are, however, other reasons to be cautious. If the equipment is not used properly, or if it is imprecise, the individual may end up inadvertently monitoring the wrong pnysiological function. Dr. Solomon Steiner of the City University of New York points out that a wide variety of facial expressions—blinking, twitching, raising of eyeballs, frowning, gritting of teeth—can produce signals quite similar to those associated with "desirable" brain wave activity. Conceivably, a person might think he is training himself to produce restful brain waves, when in actuality he is becoming a proficient twitcher.

Similar difficulties can arise, Barbara Brown points out, when the instruments or the physiological mechanisms are improperly understood. "For the most effective use of biofeedback," she writes, "it is important to know how the body expresses its emotional and mental activities through changes in its physiologic functioning." The same is true for knowledge about the procedures themselves. Studies have shown that the more information the student has about biofeedback, the better the results.

Conservative scientists point out that inadequate knowledge can lead to unanticipated difficulties, as our cavalier attitude about drugs has shown. Since we know so little about the brain, it might be penny-wise and pound-foolish to plunge helter-skelter into newer and newer applications of biofeedback before we know more about it. Evidently, very delicate neurological mechanisms are involved.

Those cautions aside, it is generally felt that biofeedback is harmless. It must, however, be done properly, under professional supervision, and only with top-notch equipment. When it was discovered that persons could train themselves to produce alpha waves, millions of people dashed out to buy biofeedback equipment. Commercial manufacturers turned out machines by the carload—often cheap, inaccurate ones. Not only was the dream of attaining euphoric states of awareness naive, but the quest proved downright dangerous.

Other questions still to be investigated include: Is the training adequately transferable to everyday life? Do patients continue to use their acquired skills when no longer under supervision? Are we relying on expensive technology for something that can be accomplished just as well without it? Do people tend to use biofeedback as a substitute for proper medical treatment?

In the meantime, a great many corporations are seriously considering the use of biofeedback equipment as an adjunct to their employee health programs. Reportedly, Xerox and Martin Marietta are keeping a close eye on research findings to see if they can use biofeedback to relax their executives and make them more creative. Shell Oil is experimenting with its uses too. NASA has already used biofeedback to train astronauts in controlling anxiety.

According to a *New York Times* report, the Equitable Life Assurance company has its own biofeedback laboratory, used by 15 to 20 employees a week, when they feel tense. James Manuso, Equitable's psychologist, estimates that every $15 spent on treatment alleviates symptoms that would otherwise have cost the company $45 in lost time or productivity.

The Hardware

In shopping for biofeedback equipment, it is important to consider the quality of the machine. Prices for portable equipment range from $300 to $800. "Although cost is usually an indicator of quality," warns Dr. Rosalind Forbes, who has used biofeedback at several large corporations, "it is not an absolute guarantee that the machine will work effectively—that it will accurately sense your muscle tension, for example, and give you correct feedback."

Dr. Elmer Green of the Menninger Foundation concurs. He tested a wide variety of commercial machines and concluded that "even the most expensive don't always work right."

Most manufacturers provide demonstration and training seminars on how to use the machines. Make sure your purchase is contingent upon the receipt of adequate personal instruction. Once purchased, make sure its use is monitored by skilled trainers and technicians.

---

information on biofeedback

The best source of information on the uses of biofeedback, places where it is taught, reliable equipment, and anything else on the subject is the Biofeedback Research Society, University of Colorado, 4200 E. 9th Avenue; Denver, Colorado 80220.

The following is a partial list of Biofeedback Centers in the United States. Consult your local telephone directory, the psychology department of a major university, or the psychiatric division of any large hospital.

New York: Maimonides Hospital in Brooklyn
Chicago: Biofeedback Clinic of Chicago
Los Angeles: Toomin Laboratories
Topeka, Kansas: The Menninger Clinic

---

the transcendental meditation technique

"From a purely financial point of view, the Transcendental Meditation program is the greatest innovation in management since the Industrial

Revolution." So says Montague Guild, Jr., president of Guild Investment Management, an international investment advisory firm. Guild should know: he has been practicing the TM technique for a dozen years. In that time, he has seen his company—and his own investment portfolio—expand "astronomically." "The longer I practiced TM, the more difficult it became to *make* mistakes," he says.

Guild's personal experience has been verified by scores of executives and entrepreneurs to whom he has taught TM in his voluntary capacity as president of the American Foundation for the Science of Creative Intelligence (AFSCI), a nonprofit organization dedicated to bringing the TM program to the business community. Greater efficiency, increased creativity, improved job performance and satisfaction, reduced absenteeism—these and a host of physical and psychological benefits have been repeatedly cited. Many have been borne out by scientific studies.

The TM technique is a simple mental practice derived from ancient Indian tradition adapted for modern Western use by the founder of the TM movement, Maharishi Mahesh Yogi, a monk, who, by virtue of his training as a physicist, amiably bridges the gap between East and West. Practicing TM involves the use of a *mantra*, a meaningless sound individually assigned to the meditator by a trained instructor. Correct use of the mantra is said to automatically reduce the level of excitation and disorderly activity of the nervous system, quieting the mind while maintaining alertness. Simultaneously, metabolic changes occur (see chart below), which point toward an extraordinarily deep state of rest.

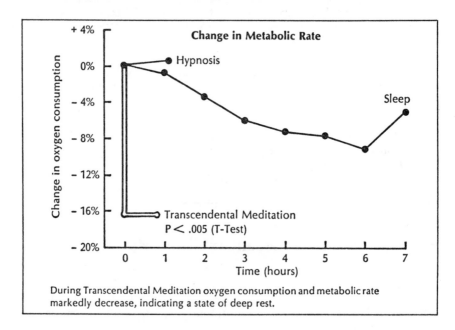

During Transcendental Meditation oxygen consumption and metabolic rate markedly decrease, indicating a state of deep rest.

Such a deep state of relaxation is what originally attracted interest in TM—it is said to enable the body to normalize the damage of stress, while at the same time strengthening the system to ward off excessive strain in the future. However, most advocates contend that TM's influence on the mind is an even more significant contribution. They claim the technique can "unfold the full conscious capacity of the mind," a reference to psychologists' belief that we use a mere fraction (5 to 15 percent) of our brain's potential.

Organizational psychologist Dr. David R. Frew concludes that for some people and in some situations, ... "Transcendental Meditation may be the single most powerful tool for dealing with the problems of organizational life...." Frew investigated TM's effects on work, expecting to find that it would reduce certain dimensions of productivity, and that meditators would find work distasteful.

But Frew's studies of 500 male and female TMers disproved his original hypotheses. He measured six variables and found the following:

Job satisfaction increased.
Performance improved.
Turnover potential was reduced (less tendency to want to switch companies).
Relationships with supervisors improved.
Relationships with co-workers improved.
Motivation to climb the corporate ladder was reduced.

Dr. Frew used self-evaluating questionnaires, but he also asked co-workers to evaluate their meditating peers. The co-workers agreed with meditators' appraisals on performance, turnover propensity, and relationships with co-workers. They agreed that the meditators' job satisfaction had improved, but not as dramatically as the meditators themselves felt it had. However, they felt that the meditators had more significantly improved their relationships with supervisors than the meditators themselves had reported.

Most meditating executives have picked up TM on their own at public courses given by the International Meditation Society, but many have taken programs specially designed for their companies by the American Foundation for the Science of Creative Intelligence. Coor's Brewing Co.; Monsanto Chemicals; Sunnydale Milk Farms; Xerox headquarters in Rochester, New York; and the Connecticut General Life Insurance Co. have all had company-sponsored TM programs set up. Some companies, such as the P.A. Medical Corporation in Tennessee, and James Sinclair & Co., a Wall Street brokerage firm, actively recruit TMers for their work force, preferring them to nonmeditators. In some cases, fringe benefits even include time off to attend TM courses.

The enthusiasm about TM among executives is apparently based on a large body of evidence. In addition to the findings already mentioned, studies have indicated that TM decreases anxiety, depression, and emotional disturbance, and increases creativity, self-reliance, memory, and perception.

One study—reported in Jay B. Marcus's *TM and Business* (McGraw-Hill 1978), investigated the effects of TM on 36 managers at a General Motors plant in Fremont, California. Nine months after instruction, a medical evaluation and a questionnaire administered by GM's personnel department turned up the following:

37% stated they needed less sleep.
50% stated they fell asleep faster.
37% stated they used less hard liquor.
23% stated they used less beer and wine (13% used more).
55% of the smokers stated they eliminated or reduced their cigarette intake.
20% stated they used less aspirin.
20% stated they used less coffee.
53% stated they are more self-confident.
60% stated they have better emotional stability.
53% stated their ability to organize had improved.

From a health point of view, physicians have lauded TM as an important preventive measure. Studies have shown that, even outside of meditation, meditators' heart and respiration rates are lower than nonmeditators'; high blood pressure tends to normalize over time; angina pectoris patients showed significant improvements in exercise tolerance and work load; bronchial asthma sufferers improved; and TM aided in weight normalization.

Perhaps most significantly, studies have also shown that meditators respond better to stress than do nonmeditators. Psychologist David Orme-Johnson studied the physiological responses to stressful stimulation (loud noxious tones) and found that meditators habituated to the stimulus faster, indicating what Orme-Johnson called "greater stability in response to stress." In addition, he found that meditators had fewer spontaneous fluctuations in skin resistance both in and out of meditation, another indication of a stable autonomic nervous system.

Is the TM Technique Unique?

TM has its detractors, of course. Some doubt the validity of many experiments cited by TM advocates, particularly those performed by advocates (who counter that they are believers *because* their experimental findings were positive, not the other way around). On the whole, however, few scientists doubt that TM does basically what its supporters claim it does. Most of the studies have withstood close scrutiny. The real point of contention is: don't other techniques do the same thing?

Early test results are mixed. It seems that other meditative techniques do produce essentially the same result—relaxation. However, it has been assumed that if another technique can duplicate one or two variables it will also produce the other results attributed to TM, and to the same degree. This may not be the case.

The initial studies on the TM technique were done in 1970 by Dr. R. K. Wallace, who later became president of Maharishi International University. Wallace described the "unique physiological correlates" he found as a "fourth major state of consciousness," qualitatively different from sleeping, dreaming, and ordinary wakefulness.

Subsequently, Wallace teamed up with Dr. Herbert Benson, a cardiologist at Harvard Medical School, who stumbled onto TM while exploring the possibility of training patients to control their blood pressure through mental volition. The pair collaborated on a series of experiments in the early 1970s, which confirmed Wallace's previous observations.

Since then, scientists have learned more about consciousness and meditation than we have in the six centuries since Marco Polo opened the doors to the Orient. The tremendous number of studies also set the stage for controversy. While often maddening to the serious inquirer, this sustained wave of scientific interest in mental states is sure to result in tremendous breakthroughs in understanding human nature and its ultimate potential.

It was Dr. Benson who—perhaps prematurely—asserted that *all* meditative and relaxation techniques produce the same set of physiologic changes. Some of these seemed to be the exact opposite of the fight-or-flight response; he labeled it the "relaxation response," and reasoned that it was a similar, natural physiological reaction. "The relaxation response appears to be an integrated hypothalamic response which results in generalized decreased sympathetic-nervous-system activity, and perhaps also increased parasympathetic activity," Benson wrote.

The notion has an aesthetic appeal to many scientists, but as Dr. Bernard Glueck, director of research at Hartford's Institute of Living, reports, "Not everyone agrees with his [Benson's] contention that humans have both an emergency response and a relaxation response system." While neurological mechanisms associated with the fight-or-flight response have been well described, it is not yet established that comparable circuits function as a relaxation mechanism.

The basic metabolic processes, however, have been reasonably well delineated, and seem to conform to Benson's contention.

Benson's conclusion that all techniques work alike, however, has stirred even more controversy. Says Dr. Glueck in *Expanding Dimensions of Consciousness* (Sugarman and Tart, eds., Springer, 1978):

> Benson argues that the built-in response systems that are designed to produce a more relaxed state within the organism are triggered by all of the relaxation techniques, be it his particular technique, Transcendental Meditation, other forms of yoga, or the increasingly sophisticated electronic approaches, using various biofeedback techniques, that are proliferating rapidly.

So far, research on similar techniques has been unable to entirely replicate the large body of data on physiology, personality, and behavior gathered on TM. One area of research unique to the TM technique has attracted considerable attention: brain wave synchrony. TMers have been found to produce more orderly (synchronous) and coherent EEG output than nonmeditators, especially balanced between the two hemispheres of the brain. Integration of left and right hemispheres could have a profound influence on creativity and decision making, researchers feel.

Experienced TM meditators also contend that virtually all simulated versions involve considerably more mental effort than TM, which is said to be natural and effortless. While other techniques do exhort the practitioner to take it easy, in actual practice the instructions are such that focusing or concentrating is virtually unavoidable. Strain can result, and the mind will not achieve much rest.

For now, it seems reasonable to assume that if meditation produces benefits, it can also work in reverse if done improperly. If there are important advantages in the formal, personal instruction of TM, then TM's worldwide network of centers, standardized teaching, follow-up procedures, and strict adherence to time-tested principles should maximize results.

TM courses cost $200 per person, with standard discounts for students and couples. In-house programs are individually designed to suit the company's needs; price varies accordingly. The basic course of instruction requires one to two hours over four consecutive days, with optional follow-up afterward. There are TM centers in every major city, and most smaller ones as well. Look up Transcendental Meditation or International Meditation Society in your phone directory. National headquarters are located at 17310 Sunset Boulevard, Pacific Palisades, Calif. 90272.

───────── **recommended reading: chapter 8** ─────────

Happiness, Bloomfield and Kory (New York: Simon & Schuster, 1976).

Management of Stress: Using TM at Work, David R. Frew (Chicago: Nelson-Hall, 1977).

New Mind, New Body, Barbara Brown (New York: Harper & Row, 1974).

Progressive Relaxation, Edmond Jacobson (Chicago: University of Chicago Press, 1938).

Relax, White and Fadiman, eds. (New York: Confucian Press, 1976).

The Massage Book, George Downing (New York: Random House, 1972).

The Psychology of Consciousness, Robert Ornstein (San Francisco: W. H. Freeman & Co., 1972).

The Relaxation Response, Herbert Benson, (New York: Morrow, 1975).

The TM Program: The Way to Fulfillment, Philip Goldberg (New York: Holt, Rinehart & Winston, 1976).

TM and Business, Jay B. Marcus (New York: McGraw-Hill, 1978).

You Must Relax, Edmond Jacobson (New York: McGraw-Hill, 1957).

a good night's sleep

---

self-evaluation: how do you sleep?

1. How long does it usually take to fall asleep?
2. Has this changed within the last year?
3. Do you awaken in the night? If so, how many times each night? How long do you remain awake?
4. Do you ever awaken prematurely, unable to return to sleep?
5. How much total sleep do you usually get? Has that changed recently?
6. Do you stay awake long after feeling sleepy?
7. Do you go to bed not feeling tired?
8. Do you wish you could remain in bed when it's time to wake up?
9. Do you take sleeping pills? How often?
10. Do you drink much alcohol in the evening?
11. Do you ever worry about whether you will sleep well?
12. Do you snore?
13. Does your spouse complain of being kicked in the night?
14. Do you do anything to aid sleep?
15. Do you bring work home with you at night?
16. Is your bedroom sufficiently quiet and dark?
17. What do you think causes your sleep problems?
18. What do you think about when lying in bed awake?
19. Do you feel you need more sleep?
20. What are your peak hours during the day?
21. What are the times of "slump"?
22. Do you ever nap during the day? Would you like to?

Sleep Log

To gain a greater awareness of your sleep patterns, problems, and needs, fill out this chart every day for two weeks. Mark the time you went to bed with an arrow pointing down, and the times you awakened with an arrow pointing up. Do this even for naps and nighttime awakenings. Mark with an * the times when falling back to sleep took more than ten minutes.

Day   Date   10P.M.   11   12   1A.M.   2A.M.. . . .

Each day, answer these questions:
1. How long did it take to fall asleep last night?
2. How often did you awaken?
3. How much total sleep did you get?
4. What time did you have to get up?
5. Was yesterday a particularly stressful day?
6. Did you have a difficult day coming up?
7. How did you feel upon awakening this morning?
8. Were you alert throughout the day?
9. Were you tired last evening?

insomnia

Watching for riches consumeth the flesh, and the care thereof driveth away sleep.—Ecclesiastes 31:1

Each night as many as 40 percent of all Americans have difficulty sleeping. Many of them are rehashing board meetings or fretting over managerial decisions. Says Dr. Elliott Goldwag, executive director of the Renaissance Revitalization Center, "Today, over 50 percent of our clients, from board chairmen to individual entrepreneurs, complain of sleep problems."

Some of them can't fall asleep upon going to bed, a condition known as *initial* insomnia. Others have *intermittent* insomnia—they wake up frequently in agitation. Still others have *matutinal* insomnia, waking up prematurely, unrefreshed, weary, and unable to fall back to sleep. In whatever form it comes, insomnia, which can be caused by any number of things, chief among which is emotional stress, can precipitate troublesome days.

The consequences of insomnia vary, depending on how much sleep is lost and on mental and physical health. An occasional rough night

Editor's Note: Some of the material in this chapter has been condensed from *Natural Sleep* (Emmaus, Pa.: Rodale Press, 1978), a comprehensive source book on insomnia by this author and Daniel Kaufman.

is relatively harmless, a quite normal reaction to a stressful day. Prolonged awakenings or consistent difficulty falling asleep, however, are the hallmarks of true insomnia, and are likely to elicit some or all of the consequences below.

---

effects of sleep loss:

dull perception
erratic and unpredictable reaction to stimuli
diminished energy level, attentiveness, memory, and task performance
impaired judgement
decreased motivation
decreased efficiency
increased hostility, depression, negativity, and apathy

If you have difficulty sleeping as much as you think you should, the first thing to do is determine how serious your problem is. The sleep log and questionnaire at the beginning of this chapter will help you understand the precise nature of your problem. It will also make you much more aware of your own sleep patterns and needs, an important step toward improving sleep.

is it really insomnia?

Many idiosyncratic sleepers have been greatly relieved to find that they actually had no problem. The following sections discuss five alternative situations that may result in *less sleep* without involving true insomnia at all.

Pseudoinsomnia

A real estate broker, forced into retirement by chronic "sleep loss," entered the sleep clinic at Stanford University. He described his sleep as fitful, estimating that he slept only five of the eight hours he spent in bed. But according to physiological recordings over two consecutive nights, he fell asleep in less than ten minutes and spent seven full hours in normal sleep.

His case is common. Says Dr. William C. Dement, director of the Stanford clinic, "Although every insomniac came to our clinic as their 'last hope' in getting some respite from the tortures of sleeplessness, the severity of their complaint had *absolutely no relation* to the amount they slept in the laboratory."

Just why poor sleepers underestimate the quality of their sleep is unknown. Some say that their sleep is so shallow it is interpreted, subjectively, as non-sleep. Others feel that time can become distorted to a person eager to sleep; two minutes awake can seem like ten or twenty. Regardless of the reason, an astonishing recovery takes place when people are told that they do, in fact, sleep normally. Relieved, they usually sleep well from then on.

Do You Really Need Eight Hours?

Many people have taken pills and gone to sleep clinics because they thought everyone is supposed to sleep a full eight hours. Actually, sleep needs are as personal as food. Napoleon, Churchill, Edison, and Goethe are only a few of history's great achievers who thrived on three to four hours of sleep a night. Even daytime fatigue might be due to factors such as diet or exercise, not the fact that you sleep less than eight hours.

Your Own Body Rhythms

Robert Brodie, regional sales manager for a major manufacturer, used to get to bed by ten, only to lie awake for two to three hours before falling asleep. Most mornings he would struggle out of bed when the alarm rang and trudge wearily to the office. Coffee and amphetamines became a way of life until a friend remarked, "Why don't you just stay up?"

Brodie tried it. He went to sleep when he felt tired rather than when the clock said he should; he fell asleep easily. Naturally, he awakened later. Consequently, he adjusted his work schedule, making no appointments before ten, and staying later at the office. He feels more alert during the day, and no longer wastes precious time awake in bed.

Many of us have internal rhythms that do not conform to society's customary timetables. Brodie was not an insomniac; he simply had an innate sleep-wake cycle that was better suited for late hours. Others are geared to an early bedtime; they would be wise to follow that inclination, perhaps beginning their work day earlier to take advantage of the freshness of morning.

Study your sleep log, and try to notice when you are most awake and when you are most inclined to sleep. Then determine the best bedtime for you and stick to it; sleep experts, unanimously advocate regularity.

jet lag

A major contributor to sleep difficulties is crossing time zones. Some executives who travel frequently are in a more or less permanent state of jet lag. Here are some tips:

If you travel constantly, try to keep your work and sleep schedules tuned to the time zone of your most frequent location, preferably home.

Plan your itinerary with room to spare. Ideally, allow one day of adjustment for every 1½ hours of time change.

If your visit is brief, schedule your meetings according to your home schedule. (ITT's New York executives start their meetings at 2:00 P.M. during their monthly board meetings in Brussels—9:00 A.M. New York time).

Start adjusting to the new time before you leave by moving your bedtime up or back each night for a few days (depending on which direction you will be traveling in).

If you are making a long trip, say to the Orient, break up the trip with a one- or two-day stopover to reset your internal clock.

Take a Nap

Some of us are better suited to a polyphasic sleep pattern—sleeping in separate stages. If you are consistently awake part of the night, get up and use the time. Then make up for it, if necessary, with a nap during the day. The nap will help alleviate the fatigue that results from a poor night's sleep and may also prevent further problems the next night.

The latter is a disputed point—some experts feel that napping interferes with normal sleep, while others feel it can help. The consensus seems to be: If you have insomnia, either nap every day or not at all.

Reportedly, the best time for a nap is right before or after lunch. "Tension increases as the day goes on," writes William Kitay in *The Challenge of Medicine.* "If the business executive breaks it at noon with a short nap the tension curve drops to near base line, and he awakens for the work of the afternoon refreshed." Some companies, like McGraw-Hill, maintain small private rooms in their infirmaries for tired employees.

Settle on a convenient time and allocate fifteen to thirty minutes for it every day. Lie down and put aside pressing problems (if they are important they will still be there when you wake up). Don't *try* to sleep. The effort might be self-defeating. Even if you do not fall asleep, fifteen minutes supine will be remarkably refreshing.

Aging

You may not have insomnia, you may just be getting older; sleep needs diminish with age. According to a report from New York's Montefiore Hospital: "Sleep efficiency decreases after thirty years in men and fifty years in women, then decreases more steeply in both sexes after the mid-fifties. The number of awakenings per night increases gradually until forty years in men and seventy years in women, then increases more steeply after those ages."

Unaware of these facts, middle-aged people often end up on sleeping pills when they stop sleeping their customary eight hours. Knowing that the change may only be a consequence of aging can alleviate the anxiety and prevent actual insomnia.

After considering these reasons for false alarms, you should be in a better position to determine whether your sleep problems are pathological. If none of these apply and your sleep patterns have changed dramatically, if the problem is persistent, and if daytime aftereffects are severe, you probably have a problem worthy of attention.

sleeping pills— hazardous and inefficient

Until recently, the first defense against insomnia was the sleeping pill. More than 100 million dollars a year is spent on sleep medication, a figure second only to aspirin sales. About thirty million doses are taken each night.

In recent years, sleep researchers have mounted an attack on the cavalier dispensation of sleeping pills. Some have advocated banning the sale of familiar products like Nytol, Dormin, Sleep-eze, and Sominex. "My feeling is, the over-the-counter sleep drugs should not be sold," said Dr. Anthony Kales, a pioneer sleep researcher. "The use and availability of these drugs are not to the advantage of the average patient."

The reason for the disenchantment is threefold:

Sleeping pills have dangerous side effects.
Sleeping pills are addictive.
Sleeping pills don't help you sleep.

Side Effects

The main ingredients in virtually all sleeping pills—antihistamine, scopolamine, or bromides—have been found to produce dangerous side effects, including kidney and liver damage, circulatory and respiratory problems, high blood pressure, central nervous system damage, impaired digestion, and a host of mental and behavioral disorders. Of bromides, a Food and Drug Administration task force reported, "The effective dose differs little from the poisonous dose."

Dalmane, the largest-selling prescription "sleeper," has caused these adverse reactions:

> *dizziness*
> *excessive drowsiness*
> *staggering*
> *loss of muscle coordination*
> *lethargy*
> *severe sedation*
> *disorientation*
> *headache*
> *heartburn*
> *nausea*
> *diarrhea*
> *vomiting*
> *constipation*
> *chest, stomach, and joint pains*
> *palpitations*
> *apprehension*
> *insomnia*

Ironically, disturbances of the nervous system can cause "drug-dependency insomnia."

Do not be fooled by claims of "safe" and "effective" on drugstore labels, doctors warn. Over-the-counter drugs are safe and effective for a few days at most.

Addiction

Virtually every "sleeper" tested loses its effectiveness within two weeks: the body develops a tolerance for it. The insomniac whose only defense is the sleeping pill typically resorts to ever-increasing dosages. The side effects multiply, as do psychological and physiological dependence. The addict will often resort to amphetamines during the day in an attempt to counteract the dullness brought on by the sleeping pills, thus creating a situation where drugs dominate the entire sleep-wake cycle.

Addiction is further compounded by the user's erroneous conviction that the pills are still helping him sleep. "The individual may, because he *believes* the drug is putting him to sleep, actually be able to relax enough so that he can doze off," states Dr. Peter Hauri, director of the sleep clinic at Dartmouth College. "But the pill isn't doing a thing. On the contrary, the pills are most probably going to disturb the pattern of his sleep."

Unlike heroin addicts, abusers of sleep medication and tranquilizers have no trouble getting what they want legitimately. Also, they are usually affluent enough to be able to afford what they need. However, social acceptability does not mask the fact that sleeping pill addiction is devastating.

---

withdrawal from sleeping pills

It is no less difficult to break a barbiturate habit than heroin addiction. Effects may include anxiety, nausea, weakness, fever, hallucinations, convulsions, twitching, delusions, hypertension, and, yes, insomnia.

Some users have withdrawn on their own using a method devised by Dr. Anthony Kales: cut out one clinical dose of the drug (the amount usually taken at night) once every week. This gradual tapering off seems to be relatively safe. However, it is best to withdraw under medical supervision. Contact your physician or a sleep clinic.

Keep in mind that one of the symptoms of withdrawl is a disturbance of sleep. This often prevents individuals from following through on their withdrawal regimen. Thinking they have had a relapse of insomnia, their first reaction is to take a pill to cure it. It takes time and perseverence to withdraw, but the benefits are worth the effort.

Disruption of Normal Sleep Patterns

Sleeping pills do not induce natural sleep—they induce narcosis, depressing the central nervous system by interfering with the passage of impulses in the brain. In the words of Dr. Edmund Jacobson, the drugs work by "delivering a knock-out blow to the brain cells. You sleep because your nerve cells are paralyzed by what you swallow." Unlike actual sleep, this is an exhaustive, rather than a recuperative process.

Significantly, sleeping pills seriously interfere with the REM stage of sleep, the stage in which a great deal of important dreaming occurs. REM sleep (for the rapid eye movements that occur in this stage) is considered vital for physical and mental health. Experiments show that persons disturbed during the REM stage develop impaired learning, memory, and performance; serious psychological disturbances; and other difficulties. They make up for the loss by "compensatory dreaming," often of a vivid, nightmarish quality, the next night.

The this reason, medical authorities are adamant about limiting the use of sleeping pills to infrequent occasions when pain or a severe crisis keeps you from falling asleep.

"If an individual is getting himself all uptight and into some sort of bind about his inability to sleep," says Dr. Peter Hauri, "and if this should continue for a few nights running, then he might be moving into a vicious cycle...." At such times, taking a pill *for one night* would not be inadvisable, as long as you are aware of the fact that you will not be getting efficient sleep, that you might feel groggy the next day, and that you will likely experience the REM rebound or compensatory dreaming the next night.

---

if you must take pills

If you ever use sleeping pills, keep these points in mind

Consult your physician; don't use over-the-counter medication unless he recommends it.

Ask what the side effects of the drug are, and if there is danger of addiction.

Never take pills after drinking: The combination can cause death.

Never take pills before driving or other tasks requiring sound mind-body coordination.

Husband and wife should not both take sleeping pills on the same night, in case of an emergency.

Dalmane, also known as Flurazapane, seems at this time to be the least dangerous of commonly used medications.

—— how to treat insomnia without drugs ——

"I think of insomnia as a symptom, not as a disease," states prominent sleep researcher Dr. Ernest Hartmann. "It is not an illness for which the sleeping pill is the cure."

Virtually all sleep experts agree. Insomnia is a sign that something is wrong—mental, physical, or behavioral factors are preventing the body from performing one of its most basic functions. Exactly how this occurs is not yet known, although researchers are zeroing in. It may have something to do with improper metabolism of serotonin, the brain chemical associated with sleep onset.

In many cases, however, the cause may be as simple as too much coffee, poor bedtime habits, or improper bedding. With chronic cases, it usually has some relation to deep-seated psychological disturbances —most insomniacs display symptoms of anxiety or depression. It can even be purely organic, a side effect of illness such as asthma, ulcers, migraine and cluster headaches, or diabetes. Angina pectoris attacks frequently occur during sleep, waking up the victim. (If you suffer from angina, do not take sleeping pills; doctors feel that REM rebound may increase the likelihood of attack, since most pains come during the REM stage.)

Stress is a major cause of insomnia. Studies have shown that increased daytime stress will lead to a decrease in stage-four sleep (the deepest stage) and to an increased number of awakenings during the REM stage. For that reason, the best way to deal with insomnia is to reduce the destructive impact of stress in your life. Several of the stress-reducing modalities already discussed have been found directly effective in improving sleep.

Exercise

"Regular exercise promotes deep sleep," writes Dr. Quentin R. Regestein, director of a Boston sleep clinic. "Insomniac patients should exercise vigorously and frequently." Regestein's view is shared by most experts; experiments have shown that vigorous physical activity in the afternoon increases the amount of time spent in stage-four sleep.

In the evening, lighter exercise is recommended—a slow swim, dancing, or a casual walk—especially for sedentary workers who need to induce some muscular fatigue without raising the metabolism too high. Using the leg muscles will help considerably. "The fatigue produced by it," claims Dr. Paul Dudley White, an enthusiastic walker, "is undoubtedly the best tranquilizer ever made, either by nature or man."

While yoga exercises are usually done during the day because they tend to boost energy, some of the postures described earlier are said to be excellent for encouraging sleep: the cobra, the neck twist, the alternate leg pull, the shoulder stand, and the corpse, in that order. Remember, slow and easy does it.

TM and Sleep

Studies have shown that insomniacs who learn the TM technique reduce their time of sleep onset by as much as 80 percent. In addition, persons deprived of sleep were able to recover more quickly if they practiced TM during the day. TM teachers recommend *not* practicing the technique before going to bed; it is, they say, a "preparation for activity," since it boosts energy and alertness. But its stress-reducing properties carry over into the night, aiding sleep.

Biofeedback

Several researchers have claimed that biofeedback training helps to relieve insomnia. "With this training," reports Dr. Thomas Budzynski of the University of Colorado, "people who had taken four hours to fall asleep were dropping into slumber twice in a twenty minute lab session."

Diet

Caffeine, of course, should be taboo for insomniacs. If you can't eliminate coffee, tea, cola, and chocolate from your diet, you should at least cut down, and you should restrict intake to the earlier part of the day. The same is true of sugar and starches, which might raise the level of arousal to the point where sleep is disturbed.

Deficiencies in calcium and the B vitamins have been connected to insomnia. Orthomolecular psychiatrists claim success in treating poor sleepers with large doses of niacinamide, a B vitamin.

Overeating at night, particularly heavy foods, is another contributing factor—if the body is digesting an overload, it cannot settle down properly.

Snoring

On any given night, as many as twenty-five million Americans snore. It is no laughing matter—not for those kept awake listening, nor for those doing the snoring.

In some cases, snoring can be caused by nasal obstructions created by enlarged adenoids, tonsils, polyps, allergies, or excessive smoking. It occurs most often when lying on the back, when the back of the tongue might fall against the throat walls causing the tongue and throat tissues to vibrate.

---

snoring

If your snoring is not related to apnea, or to any other physical defect, here are some techniques to help cure it:

Have your spouse wake you up when you begin to snore, perhaps by rigging up a buzzer. That will help break the habit.

Don't sleep on your back. Try sleeping on your side with your forearm under your chin to keep your mouth closed. Place pillows behind you to prevent rolling over onto your back.

Attach a small ball to the back of your pajamas to discourage sleeping on your back.

Increase the humidity in your room; dry membranes swell, sometimes increasing snoring.

Lose weight; obese persons snore more.

If nasal obstruction is present, check with your doctor for nose drops, sprays, or other decongestants.

Recommended reading: How To Stop Snoring, *by David Harwich.*

Your Evening Routine

"Going to sleep is like stopping a car at an intersection," writes Dr. Dean Foster, consultant to the Sleep Research Foundation. "A driver who sees a traffic light change a block away is better off slowing down gradually and coasting to a stop, rather than coming to a sudden, brake-slamming halt. Taper off your day's activities before getting ready for bed."

going to bed

If you have insomnia, start preparing for bed when you leave the office. Don't take work home with you; if you must work, stop at least an hour before bedtime.

Don't get too keyed up at night and don't persist in a task once you are exhausted.

Reserve evenings for light activities. Reading material should be unrelated to work, and not too stimulating. Save movies, TV, or theater for the weekend, keeping mid-week entertainment simple and pleasant.

Save heavy discussions, especially arguments, for the early part of the evening; if possible, conclude them—nothing is worse than stewing over all the things you should have said.

Keep musical fare soothing, not invigorating. Try the Goldberg Variations, *by J. S. Bach (written to lull an insomniac patron to sleep).*

Get to bed as soon as you feel sleepy. Don't fight it: you may win.

Accent protein and calcium foods in the evening. Dairy products, particularly easily digested ones like cottage cheese, are excellent. Stay away from junk-food snacks.

A glass of warm milk before bed may be more than an old wive's tale.
It has calcium, protein, and l-tryptophane (see "Sleep Inducers,"
below). Add honey, Postum, or Ovaltine for flavor.
Chamomile tea is a natural sedative.
Use alcohol sparingly. It can suppress dreams and make sleep more
fitful. A four-ounce glass of wine half an hour before bed is said
to help produce drowsiness.
Take a warm bath: the water should be between ninety and one hun-
dred degrees. Add baking soda, oil of eucalyptus, or mustard pow-
der. Immerse up to your neck, dim the lights, close your eyes, and
unwind. Soak until the water cools, pat yourself dry, and get right
to bed.

Once You Are in Bed

Your room should be quiet. If it is not that way, and if noise bothers you, try ear plugs. Flents, Inc. makes a wax type that can be purchased inexpensively in any pharmacy. A favorite in industry is the E-A-R plug, made by Time and Space Enterprises in Hollywood, California. They are made of a polymer that expands to conform to the contours of any ear. Don't use the type of plugs meant for swimmers.

Some people prefer unobtrusive, repetitive sounds to silence. A device called Marsona, manufactured by the Marpac Company of Wilmington, Delaware, electronically produces the lulling sounds of rain, wind, and surf. It comes with volume control and is designed for continuous operation.

For those whose bedrooms are impossible to darken adequately, a good pair of eyeshades can come in handy. There is even one with tiny pinholes for those who like it dark but not too dark.

These and dozens of other sleep gadgets can be obtained in specialty shops like Hammacher-Schlemmer in New York. Perhaps the best source of information on sleep-aids is Mr. Norman Dine, who has been dubbed "America's Public Sandman," and has been servicing insomniacs for over forty years. Write for a catalogue: 33 Halsted Street, East Orange, New Jersey.

Your Bed

Unromantic as it may sound, single beds are recommended for insomniacs. Writes Dr. P. J. Steincrohn: "There is more likelihood of loss of sleep and consequent irritability and argument in double beds than in twin beds (no elbows in the ribs, no twisting and turning)."

beds

Most orthopedists suggest firm mattresses. Dr. Leon Root, coauthor of
Oh, My Aching Back, *recommends a hard, foam mattress, four to
six inches thick, on an inch-thick plywood board. Your bed can be
too firm, however. If you feel pressure at the hips or other heavy
parts of the body, and if your mobility is limited, that might be
the case.*

*Mattresses should be eight to ten inches longer than you are, and
seven to ten inches wider, in order to facilitate movement (we
shift position up to fifty times per night).*

*When choosing a mattress, lie down on it. Find one that provides a
bouyant, cradling sensation, complete freedom of movement, and
evenly distributed pressure.*

*Your pillow should be just thick enough to hold the head in a straight
line with the spine.*

*The best temperature for sleep is said to be between 60 and 65 degrees.
Experts recommend well-ventilated rooms. With the aid of electric blankets, down comforters, foot warmers, and other devices
you should be able to find the right combination of fresh air and
warmth.*

*The "ideal" position for sleep is with spine straight, knees and elbows
relaxed, limbs away from the body, shoulders and hips anchored.
It may take some getting used to—don't strain, just ease into this
position whenever you are aware of lying on your back or stomach.*

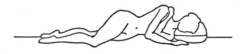

How to Coax Sleep

"Sleep ought not to have to be enticed like a frightened fawn," wrote
English author Arnold Bennett. "It should pounce on you like a tiger."
Here are some tips for setting an enticing trap.

TAKE YOUR SPOUSE TO BED, NOT YOUR PROBLEMS States psy-
chiatrist-author David Viscott: "At bedtime, when perspective is
slanted to begin with because defenses are altered, you can't deal with
problems positively. So you shouldn't deal with them at all.... Remember, you probably already know everything you need to solve your
problems in the morning.... You need rest, not knowledge."

DON'T WORRY Without strain, and without becoming a psychic ostrich, turn your attention to positive thoughts. Think back to pleasant memories or times when you overcame the type of problem that now confronts you. Fears are easily exaggerated in the still of the night.

DON'T WORRY ABOUT INSOMNIA Fear of not sleeping is a leading cause of sleeplessness. Studies have shown that sleep-deprived individuals function remarkably well the next day, *if* they are strongly motivated. Your body will not tolerate sleeplessness very long; ultimately, it will conk out, and you will recover from prior deprivation quickly.

DON'T TRY TO SLEEP Sleep is a quiescent state; the act of trying is an excited state. Effort, however simple, will keep the brain engaged just when it should be in neutral.

MIND GAMES If done without effort, they can keep your mind on cheerful distractions when it might otherwise get caught up in worry. Imagine an idyllic scene, recall fond memories, spell words backward, name cities or countries from A to Z, plot a drive across the country, cast a movie of your life with Hollywood stars.

——————— some proven sleep inducers ———————

If you are able to reduce the negative impact of stress in your waking life, you should, ideally, fall asleep soon after hitting the pillow. If, however, sleep does not come within fifteen minutes or so, or if you awaken agitated and unable to fall back asleep, try one of these simple techniques.

The Kelly Method

Developed by Dr. Charles Kelly, this breathing technique is designed to increase the carbon dioxide level in the blood, which is conducive to sleep.

> *Lie either on your back or side, using a pillow that keeps your head straight or slightly tilted backward (don't lean the head forward). Eyes closed, breathe deeply, filling the lungs as much as possible. Exhale fully, drawing in the abdomen to expel as much air as possible. Repeat this three times. After the third exhalation, hold the breath as long as you can.*

Repeat the entire procedure (three breaths per set) five times. You should feel relaxed by then. If you are drowsy sooner, stop and allow yourself to drift into sleep.

If, once you have mastered the technique, sleep still does not come, increase to eight repetitions. If it still does not work, try this variation:

Again, take three deep breaths and maximum exhalations.
After the third, instead of holding the breath, breath in and out so slightly that the movement of air in the nostrils is barely perceptible. Each breath should be very short.
During this "minimum breathing" period, don't try to fill the lungs, and don't tense your muscles. Remain relaxed.
Perform minimum breathing until you feel the urge to breathe more deeply. Then start another series of three deep breaths, again doing minimum breathing afterwards.
Continue in this manner as long as necessary, and as long as it is comfortable, taking periods of normal breathing in between repetitions.

Do not strain during this breathing practice. If your mind drifts, don't try to remain alert; remember, you are doing this to fall asleep. Stop any time you feel like dozing off.

The Steincrohn Method

Developed by Dr. Peter Steincrohn, this technique is designed to reduce muscular tension, a major enemy of sleep.

Lying on your back, clench your left fist tightly. Raise your arm off the bed, with all muscles tensed. Hold for about a minute, then let the arm go suddenly limp. Repeat with the other arm.
Push both toes downward as far as they will go. Hold for a minute, then release the tension.
Repeat the arm and toe procedures, this time relaxing the muscles gradually instead of suddenly.
Relax your chest by taking a deep breath, holding it, and letting it go suddenly limp. Repeat with gradual relaxing.
Raise your eyebrows, thus tensing the forehead muscles. Let go. Frown, then let go. Repeat, relaxing gradually.
Eyes still closed, look as far as you can to the right and hold for half a minute. Relax. Repeat, looking to the left. Look up toward the hairline, hold, and relax. Look toward your chin, hold, and relax.
Count out loud to ten. Notice the tension in the throat, lips, tongue, and face. Relax all those muscles. Repeat the count, speaking softer

> *and softer. Now do it without using the speech muscles. Relax the entire face.*

According to Dr. Steincrohn, regular practice should eventually result in the ability to trigger overall relaxation at will.

Get Out of Bed

The bed is for sleeping in. According to Dr. Peter Hauri, many persons who have insomnia come to hate the night because they dread being unable to sleep. That fear may become self-fulfilling. "In this kind of case," says Dr. Hauri, "the individual has, somewhere along the line, become conditioned to his bedtime environment. The pillow, the bed, the lamp, etc., are not cues for drowsiness but for increased alertness and arousal. And so he starts tossing and turning."

It becomes, then, a matter of reconditioning. Dr. Richard E. Bootzin of Northwestern University has devised a behavioral modification approach, deceptively simple, for overcoming what he calls "misuse of bed."

> *Go to bed only when you are tired.*
> *Get out of bed if sleep does not come in ten minutes.*
> *Leave the room entirely at that time; the bed is not for rumination, it is for sleep.*
> *Return to the bedroom only when you think you can fall asleep.*
> *If sleep again does not come in ten minutes, get out of the room.*
> *Continue in this way through the night, never remaining in bed more than ten minutes under any circumstance.*
> *Set the alarm for the same time every day, including weekends.*
> *Never oversleep, even if you have only fallen asleep minutes before the alarm goes off.*

Needless to say, this reconditioning procedure takes a good deal of fortitude. Reportedly, the first few nights are torture. The person will typically remain awake most of the night. But within a week he may only be awake for an hour or two. Within about two or three weeks, Hauri says, "many chronic insomniacs can be retrained."

L-Tryptophane: The Safe Sedative

Perhaps the most important breakthrough in the search for natural, safe methods of aiding sleep has been the discovery of the amino acid l-tryptophane.

Found in milk (thus lending credence to warm milk as a soporific), meats, fish, poultry, eggs, nuts, soybeans, and other protein-rich foods, l-tryptophane is an essential amino acid that takes part in a number of metabolic processes, the most significant of which is the production of serotonin, the so-called sleep juice.

Dr. Ernest Hartmann, director of the sleep clinic at Boston State Hospital, has conducted research on l-tryptophane for a number of years. "In our studies," he reports, "we found that a dose of one gram of tryptophane will cut down the time it takes to fall asleep from 20 to 10 minutes. Its great advantage is that not only do you get to sleep sooner, but you do so without the distortions in sleep patterns that are produced by most sleeping pills."

A series of eleven studies led Dr. Hartmann to conclude that trypto-phane "reduces sleep latency, and usually reduces waking time." He also reports that the patients "described the effects as an increase in normal tiredness—they were seldom 'knocked out.'"

Significantly, tryptophane is not a drug that works by depressing the central nervous system. It is a nutritional substance, one or two grams of which is taken in through a normal daily diet. So far, no side effects have been found, even when high dosage has been administered over a period of months. However, doctors fear that insomniacs might tend to use tryptophane as a crutch, ignoring the underlying physical or emotional problems that are causing their sleep problems. Judicious use is recommended.

In addition to eating those protein-rich foods that contain l-trypto-phane, especially in the evening, supplements may be obtained. While it is a rare pharmacy that carries tryptophane, most well-stocked health food stores can get it for you. Dr. Hartmann recommends one gram twenty minutes before bedtime.

sleep clinics

Scientific interest in sleep began in earnest about a decade ago. The initial emphasis was on research, but that soon led to a mushrooming of treatment centers. Most of these centers are staffed by physicians, psychiatrists, psychologists, neurologists, and other specialists, and are equipped with sophisticated technology to record brain wave patterns and other physiological processes. Called polysomnograms, these recordings permit the scrupulous diagnoses that determine each individual's treatment.

Should you go to a clinic? "If the patient is a chronic insomniac," says Dr. Elliot Weitzman, director of the center at Montefiore Hospital in New York, "and it's not something that just comes and goes, he should see a physician. If he is not satisfied, if it does not solve the problem, then he should be seen in a clinic."

directory of sleep clinics

City	Address	Director
Atlanta, Ga.	Emory University School of Medicine	Dr. Gerald Vogel
Boston, Mass.	Boston State Hospital 591 Morton Street	Dr. Ernest Hartmann
Boston, Mass.	Peter Brent Brigham Hospital	Dr. Quentin Regestein
Cincinnati, Ohio	Christian R. Holmes Hospital University and Bethesda Avenues	University of Cincinnati
Cincinnati, Ohio	Veteran's Administration Hospital	Dr. Milton Kramer
Columbus, Ohio	Ohio State University Dept. of Psychiatry	Dr. Helmut Schmidt
Hanover, N.H.	Dartmouth College Medical School	Dr. Peter Hauri
Hershey, Pa.	Pennsylvania State University Milton S. Hershey Medical Center	Dr. Anthony Kales
Houston, Texas	Baylor College of Medicine	Dr. Ismet Karacan
Los Angeles, Calif.	Southern Calif. Center for Sleep Disorders 1260 15th Street Santa Monica, Calif.	Dr. John Beck
Memphis, Tenn.	Neurophysiology Laboratory Baptist Memorial Hospital	Dr. H. Lemmi
New York, N.Y.	Montefiore Hospital 111 E. 210th Street Bronx, N.Y.	Dr. Elliot Weitzman
Oklahoma City, Oklahoma	Veteran's Administration Hospital 921 N.E. 13th Street	Dr. William C. Orr
Pittsburgh, Pa.	Western Psychiatric Institute 3811 O'Hara Street	Dr. David Kupfer
San Diego, Calif.	Veteran's Administration Hospital 3350 La Jolla Village Drive	Dr. Daniel Kripke
San Francisco, Calif.	University of California School of Medicine	Dr. Jean-Paul Spire
Stanford, Calif.	Stanford University Medical Center	Dr. William C. Dement

Experts agree that the great majority of cases can be self-treated, or treated by the average physician or psychologist. Clinics should be facilities of last resort. However, some disorders—often related to insomnia—can only be diagnosed in a sleep clinic. If you have a tendency to snore heavily, especially if you are over forty and overweight, and if daytime sleepiness is a chronic problem, you may have *apnea,* a breathing obstruction that interferes with sleep.

Similarly, if your spouse complains of being kicked in the night, and if you have leg jitters—difficulty keeping your leg still while lying in bed awake—then *nocturnal myoclonus* is a possible diagnosis. In both cases, polysomnograms will either confirm or refute the possibility.

At most major sleep centers, you will be given a complete physical, a neurological exam, and a psychiatric interview. Then your sleep will be recorded for two consecutive nights. The data will be analyzed by technicians, interpreted by physicians, and discussed by the team. A treatment regimen will then be prescribed.

The fee schedule at Montefiore, a typical one, is $150 for initial evaluation; eight-hour polysomnogram, $200; each additional polysomnogram, $100; psychiatric consultation, if necessary, $100; and additional fees depending on the individual case.

───────── **recommended reading: chapter 9** ─────────

Insomnia, Luce and Segal (New York: Doubleday, 1969).

Insomniacs of the World, Goodnight! Hilary Rubinstein (New York: Random House, 1974).

Natural Sleep: How to Get Your Share, Goldberg and Kaufman (Emmaus, Pa.: Rodale Press, 1978).

The Functions of Sleep, Ernest Hartmann (New Haven, Conn.: Yale University Press, 1973).

lifestyle:
healthy
management at
work and at
home

———————————— the turn toward the individual ————————————

In October 1977, AT&T began a series of Corporate Policy Seminars entitled "The Shaping of Tomorrow." In groups of 48, 1700 executives attended the week-long programs "to prepare the top managers of the Bell System to anticipate and deal imaginatively with the changing expectations of society."

The week-long intensive—interspersed with free time for skiing, tennis, personal development, and other elective activities—called upon outside experts to cover such topics as:

"Prospects for the Future," an analysis of alternative socioeconomic futures;
"New Dimensions in Political Power," an analysis of government, mass media, consumerism, and other forms of group power;
"The Marketplace of the Future," an investigation of shifting objectives and priorities within society; and
"The Changing Nature of Work and Workers," an examination of new attitudes and expectations about work.

AT&T hopes the participants will emerge from the seminar with an enlarged perspective, along with greater flexibility, creativity, and responsiveness to social forces. AT&T is, in effect, recognizing that the modern executive must deal with faster change and greater complexity

239

than ever before. By helping its managers do so, the company is not only making them better executives, but healthier ones as well.

Such programs are becoming increasingly common. So, too, are programs directly aimed at stress management, as executives seek ways to counteract overloads engendered by the work environment. About 70 percent of our time is spent at work or in work-related activities such as commuting. Our psychic investment is even more significant; we measure each other's worth largely by our respective vocations.

Furthermore, work provides sources of satisfaction far beyond social status or economic considerations. As perhaps our chief form of self-expression, work is a psychological and emotional necessity so powerful that—despite rampant job dissatisfaction—surveys repeatedly show the overwhelming majority of people preferring to work even if all material needs were satisfied.

---

a stress management program at a large corporation

Kaiser-Permanente, a prototypical health maintenance organization (HMO), is currently experimenting with a stress prevention plan for staff at its Los Angeles Medical Center.

The pilot program was developed by Sally Nelson, a private therapist, and Don Isbell, a registered nurse and psychiatric liaison at Kaiser-Permanente, in conjunction with Dr. Mitchell Klionsky. So far it has been given to a group of nursing directors and supervisors, a group of middle-level managers, and a mixed group of physicians and nurses.

The program takes place over four consecutive days (eight hours twice and four hours twice), and combines educational and experiential components; it focuses on two principal sources of stress—intrapersonal (arising from within the individual) and interpersonal.

In lectures and seminars, participants are given a basic understanding of the mechanics of stress, its sources, and its consequences. Principles of illness prevention are communicated, and the group is taught relaxation and breathing techniques to lower "the stress response threshold." Assertion training, role playing, and psychodrama are included in intensive workshops.

Each member is given an "unstress tool kit," including cassette tapes with relaxation instructions, a Stress Symptom Checklist, and materials for constructing their own stress profiles. Participants keep daily stress journals, recording situations that arouse stress, the symptoms invoked, and other factors. Instructions are provided for scoring, and after learning stress management procedures, their effectiveness is also scored.

Journals are kept four weeks following the workshops; then the group meets in a follow-up session to review material learned, ask questions, and share reactions to the program.

Thus, for both corporate benefit and that of the employees, those who shape the way men and women spend their working hours have begun to think seriously about the human side of work. To many, it is clear that the work milieu should be as conducive as possible to growth and happiness, and certainly not destructive to those goals.

the impact of modern theories of management

For centuries, the prevailing belief has been that work is synonymous with *toil*. Ronald D. Barnes, a business consultant formerly with the Menninger Foundation, feels that up to 90 percent of the population now spends their time and energy at jobs that do not advance their own lifegoals.

Modern individuals are becoming much less willing to spend the majority of their time at unsatisfying, or even life-damaging, pursuits. *New York Times* writer Kathy Slobogin, in her article on executive stress, summed it up well:

> The values of the 1960s may be out of fashion to the extent that it's no longer considered unattractive or reactionary to be ambitious and to want power and wealth, but one lesson of the 1960s that has taken hold is that ambition, power, and wealth aren't enough, and that some measure of serenity is desirable and even necessary to survive.

From Theory X to Theory Y

The authoritarian or autocratic approach is associated with "Theory X," after the work of Douglas McGregor, professor of industrial management at MIT. The "average individual" is viewed as lacking in ambition, disliking responsibility, resisting change, and being selfish, unconcerned with the welfare of the company, and determined to work as little as possible. Traditionally, authoritarian management used familiar tactics to motivate employees—cajoling, persuading, rewarding, and punishing; tasks were rigidly delineated, carefully controlled, and closely directed.

In the late 1930s and early 1940s, the famous Hawthorne Studies found that paying attention to employees, listening to their problems, and showing an interest in them as individuals significantly increased productivity. Technical changes designed to improve efficiency turned out to be less successful than the human touch.

This realization helped bring about the human relations approach to management, which received strong backing from experts like McGregor, Chris Argyris, Rensis Likert, and Frederick Hertzberg, along with considerable opposition from classical theorists. The argument continues, but the humanists are winning.

McGregor felt that Theory X failed to acknowledge both the higher needs of human beings and their innate potential for self-development. As a result, management policies associated with Theory X could not elicit a high degree of motivation or satisfaction. McGregor's alternative Theory Y credits people with innate tendencies toward self-expression, readiness to assume responsiblity, and the ability to reconcile their own and their organization's goals.

In McGregor's view, management's responsibility was to make it possible for employees to develop their own inner potential. By so doing, the worker gained satisfaction and the company gained productivity.

Despite widespread acceptance of evolving theories, change has come slowly. It requires a lot of capital and a lot of risk to revamp organizational structure to the degree called for by proponents of the human relations school. It also takes wisdom. No one quite knows how to implement organizational changes to produce the desired results; nor does one procedure work for all people or all organizations.

Management by Objectives (MBO), for example, wherein the work group sets its own goals, has gained acceptance and considerable use. But MBO and similar procedures have not always worked. The conclusion now emerging from the ongoing debate between classical theorists and human relations theorists is that the style of management should be determined largely by the nature of the task.

"human relations" and "classical" organizational structure

Democratic	*Autocratic*
1. Informal, participative, flexible	Formal; reliance on authority, inflexible
2. No hierarchy; multidirectional communication	Rigid hierarchy; downward communication with decisions made at the top
3. Generalized functions, with each department having a broad view	Specialization, with standardized breakdown of functions. Emphasis on routine
4. Motivation is self-directed, and the emphasis is on participatory decision making. The person, rather than the task, is the important factor	Emphasis is on acting in accord with the rules, and the accomplishment of the task.

Democratic vs. Autocratic Management

It is perhaps congenial to the egalitarian spirit of our age to advocate the democratic model. But anyone who has seen an organization try to maintain efficiency in an overly democratic environment knows that all too often chaos ensues. With the other extreme, stale, rigid thinking and widespread dissatisfaction ensue. Thus, most organizations are somewhere in the middle.

Recently, Paul Lawrence and Jay Lorsch of Harvard Business School defined the criteria for preferring either the autocratic or the democratic mode. Contingency theory, as it has come to be known, is summed up by Dr. David Frew:

> Simple, predictable tasks with short-time perspectives ought to be approached with a classical management perspective. Conversely, complex, dynamic, and unpredictable tasks should employ a more democratic or human-relations approach. Tasks which are judged to be somewhat between highly complex and simple require a middle approach.

The conclusion is that managers should be flexible, and fit their style to the task and people at hand. By so doing, not only is efficiency improved, but a good deal of stress is eliminated through avoiding the conflicts that arise when policies, relationships, or personnel—either leaders or followers—are inappropriate to the task at hand.

Democratization

While it is clear that neither extreme will be universally effective, contingency theory strongly suggests the need for increased democratization of the work environment. Not only are modern individuals less willing to submit blindly to authority, but the world of work is becoming more complex. More and more organizations, and departments within organizations, are discovering that adherence to rigid boundaries is both deadening to the spirit and counterproductive. Managers, especially, need breathing room to be imaginative.

Writes Richard Cornuelle, a former executive vice-president of the National Association of Manufacturers, in *De-Managing America:* "Highly structured, authoritarian, bureaucratic organizations were able to function passably well in a simpler world. But they cannot keep up with change. They cannot digest diversity, and our society is becoming almost incomprehensibly diverse."

Cornuelle holds to the extreme position that organizations, and society as a whole, are effective *despite* the attempts of front-office management to control things, not because of it. "Businessmen tend to accept the Jeffersonian proposition that governments govern best when they govern least," he notes sardonically. "But they reject its corollary; that companies manage best when they manage least." He pleads for leadership style that will emancipate the innate creativity of even the humblest assembly-line worker by specifying *goals* instead of *behavior*. Management, he feels, could be a science only if the managees were inanimate objects, but human qualities are not subject to precise and permanent definitions. "You can command a man to turn a nut on an assembly line," says Cornuelle, "but you cannot command him to be creative or concerned or resourceful."

To the degree, therefore, that the modern world requires us to deal with uncertainty, unpredictability, and rapid change, it would seem that it is incumbent upon management to lean in the direction of the human relations approach without sacrificing the efficiency and security that a certain amount of autocracy provides. The degree to which the two are fused should, apparently, be determined by the nature of the task.

current applications in management

The health and success of individuals in the world of work is largely determined by the degree to which their human needs for dignity, self-expression, and growth are met.

Task Assignment

Management consultant Christopher Hegerty feels that prevalent management principles are backward. "The thrust is to catch people doing wrong and come down on them," he says. "We should look for right behavior and reward it." Through poor communication and egocentric behavior, Hegerty maintains, managers often create resentment and indifference among subordinates. The stress produced is deadening to health and productivity. The answer, says Hegerty, is trust.

"Most people most often live *up* to the level to which they are trusted," goes the Hegerty tenet, "or *down* to the level to which they are distrusted." His "vital tasks management," which he claims reduces boredom and resentment, relies on trust but is not overly romantic: "Trust must be established carefully and responsibly. Vital tasks management is not promiscuous love in management."

Here are the seven steps in Hegerty's vital tasks management, reprinted with permission from the author:

Step One   The manager looks at each position that reports to him and identifies the specific identifiable tasks each of the persons could do to perfrom the job with excellence. The manager makes a list of these in clear language.

Step Two   The manager then has each of the persons look at his/her own specific job and identify his or her perception of the specific tasks that would cause him or her to do the job with excellence. The managee makes a list of these in clear language.

Step Three   The manager and the managees (individually) then merge the two lists through negotiation, *not imposition.* The result is that each person now has his/her own *vital tasks agenda.*

Step Four   The managee then grades his/her own performance against the Vital Tasks Agenda and gives his/her self-evaluation of his/her job to the manager *regularly* and *frequently.*

Step Five   The manager reviews the evaluation, with each person, *never criticizing.* In the areas where the person is performing poorly, the manager asks how he/she is going to improve his/her performance. The manager listens *to* each person carefully and, if asked, offers suggestions. He does *not impose solutions!*

Step Six   Each person then uses his/her ingenuity and experiments with different strategies to improve the tasks where performance is lacking.

Step Seven   The manager then does a Vital Tasks Agenda for his/her own job and evaluates his/her own performance regularly and frequently.

©C. J. Hegarty & Co. P.O. Box 1152, Novato, Calif. 94947. 1977 Reprinted with permission from the author. All Rights Reserved.

Control of Space and Time

One of the most important results of stress research is the discovery that control over one's environment is a key factor in determining the degree of stress encountered. That, plus the demands of an increasingly complex world, had led many companies to grant greater flexibility to staff.

New York magazine writer T. George Harris, reporting on the environmental research of psychologist Robert Sommer, states: "In prisons, classrooms, offices, and college dorms, he had found again and again that such symbolic freedoms as the right to paint your own wall, whatever color, helps turn institutional space into personal space."

It seems that morale, job satisfaction, and even performance rise when persons are provided with privacy in which to work, or when they are consulted on the design of the work space. Harris reports that architects and designers may, in the future, "work as consultant to the actual users of office space, rather than pushing on with their snobs' role as builders of monuments to themselves and as promoters for the hard-edged image of corporate clients."

Flexitime

The new freedom has cut into the classical 9-to-5 day. Stimulated by the entry into the work force of women who must also attend to the needs of their families, an estimated 3000 American firms and half a million employees are now on *flexitime,* the system that enables executives and assembly-line workers alike to come and go at times of their own choosing.

Flexitime was first tried by a West German aerospace company in 1967. Since then its use has spread widely in the United States: such companies as Control Data, General Motors, National Cash Register, Nestle, American Airlines, and Pacific Gas & Electric are using it with good results.

One of the first companies to use flexitime was Montgomery Ward's New York-based Wearing Apparel and Buying Office. "Punctuality has significantly improved," says personnel manager W. J. Hughes, quoted in *Ambassador* magazine (December 1977). "There is group pressure to adhere to the schedule." He reports that everyone has responded favorably, even "old-time department managers who predicted dire consequences."

Fears of communication breakdowns, unattended offices, and outright anarchy have turned out to be unfounded. Managers at Metropolitan Life Insurance Co., where 400 employees experimented with flexitime, noted increased productivity and decreased absenteeism and tardiness. Similarly, a year-long SmithKline Corp. study of 175 employees in Philadelphia found that turnover, tardiness, and absenteeism decreased—the last by a third—at the same time that overtime dropped sharply.

There are several variations of flexitime. The most common provides for "core hours" when everyone must work. This, of course, insures adequate communication and coordination of activities. In some cases, employees are allowed to carry over a certain number of hours from month to month, the total number of weekly or monthly hours being required to average out to the customary 35 or 40 per week.

Some companies have gone even further, allowing workers access to the company at all hours, or assigning tasks with no time requirement—an employee can do his job whenever it suits him, providing he meets the deadline and performs adequately. Such extremes, of course, are not always possible or desirable.

Flexitime, it is said, makes employees feel more in control, more human, and better able to balance their personal commitments with their work. They don't have to lose pay or vacation time to get a tooth filled; nor do they need to have a stranger dress and feed their children. Employees are responding with greater efficiency and responsibility. Flexitime may well be corroborating the Theory Y school of thought. But the most significant contribution of flexitime in health terms is the mutual trust it creates between management and employees which should cut down considerably on interpersonal tension.

career compatibility and work style

The organizational chart that spells out lines of authority and communication has come to symbolize the rigid bureaucracy that came into being when small-scale entrepreneurship was replaced by the multilayered corporation. Until recently, it was assumed that adherence to the chart is necessary for cohesion and efficiency, without which a company would resemble a beehive under attack.

As with other sacred notions, this too has been forced to evolve by complex and rapidly changing modern business needs. In companies that have torn down the chart, executives feel they can make adjustments in manpower or procedures without requiring major changes in the organization ranks.

"Some people are bigger than their squares, others fill them only halfway," says David Newcomb, president of Buffalo Forge. "We don't need a chart here simply because our eye is on the project or problem, not on the position; and we understand the talents of the different people who work here and where they best fit."

Duido Ruicci, president of Horst Manufacturing Co., is quoted in *40,* a publication for chief executive officers: "Once a man is tied to a block on the organization chart, the man has to do what's on it. He has to play a role. If he weren't there, he might pick up a ball in another man's court without worrying about going through channels—and help out the company."

While most companies would not flirt with the hazards of tearing up the organization chart entirely (in many cases ambiguity of roles would lead to large-scale insecurity or confusion) many are finding new ways to get around the strict adherence to predetermined roles. Some try to go both ways, trading off the efficiency of the bureaucracy with the creativity of looser structures.

In some companies, task forces focused on particular problems constantly bring together talent from divergent divisions and levels of authority. Other companies have regular brainstorming sessions in which representatives from different departments are encouraged to leave their titles behind. Others attempt cross-pollination of ideas by openly encouraging disagreement and the use of invisible lines of communication.

Decentralization of authority is also gaining favor, particularly in conglomerates and companies with several product lines. Autonomy within each unit fosters the fertile flow of ideas and gives individuals greater control over their work. While done solely in the name of productivity, such developments should have a significant impact on health by reducing sources of potential distress.

Fit the Job to the Person

The job-personality fit, most experts feel, is essential to both productivity and health. Nothing is more stressful than laboring eight hours a day at work that is unsuited to you; that goes for owners, chief executives, and rank-and-file alike.

"Money, status, security, career, and promotion opportunity all provide random and complex inducements for the individual to take certain jobs," writes Dr. Frew, "But neither these criteria nor the typical organization itself is tuned into the most important question: What are the psychological needs of the worker?" Does he thrive on challenge, change, variety? Or does he need the comfort and security of predictability? Does she excel at complex, long-term assignments for which she has carte blanche? Or does she require simple, short-range tasks with highly structured instructions? Is he a loner, or someone who thrives on teamwork?

Surprisingly, most experts agree that managers, when considering promotions and new assignments, give too much weight to education, skills, experience, and customary career tracks—but not enough to psychological factors. The result is a lot of people working at jobs for which they are psychologically ill suited, a detriment to the company and a major source of distress for the individual. Writes Dr. Sidney Lecker:

> The biggest problem I see in the work setting is the mismatch between the personality style and the task. If you take somebody who is really good on a one-to-one level and stick him in a group, he is going to buckle under. Or if he's a group person who thrives on social stimulation and he's put off into an isolated research situation he can go crazy. The work may be a good step forward in his career, but the psychological environment is toxic.

Lecker sees the goal of matching job to personality occurring in business in two ways. The first involves helping to equip the employee with the psychological skills needed for a particular job. Suppose, for example, you have a compulsive person who hates loose ends, and hates dealing with large numbers of people at the same time, who is promoted to a supervisory position involving just those conditions. He should be prepared to handle it, with the help of a psychologist if necessary.

The second step is to get executives to consult with behavioral specialists before making key decisions where psychological factors are central; or to equip executives with the sensitivity and skills to match jobs to personalities. Right now such insight belongs only to the "intuitive psychologists" among executives, and they are the exception.

Your Style as Leader and Follower

Your degree of happiness at work may be largely determined by the degree to which your style of functioning matches your job. The questionnaire on pages 250–255 can be used to stimulate your thinking about your leadership and followership roles within your organization. In addition, it can provide useful insight into your subordinates. Do their followership styles match your leadership style and the degree of complexity of the task? Can you adapt your leadership style according to the nature of the task? Such an instrument might help you determine job or procedural suitability, which directly affect the health of yourself, your employees, and your company.

Changing Careers

The work, of course, should not only be suited to your personality, it should also be enjoyable: it may even be essential. "To achieve peace of mind and fulfillment through self-expression," writes Dr. Selye, "most men need a commitment to work in the service of some cause that they can respect."

The burgeoning executive recruitment business is indicative of the increase in executive mobility. Not only are companies poking around the ranks of rival companies with all the determination of college football scouts, but the onus of having switched companies is no longer the detriment it once was. Companies like it when other companies do their training for them. Executive mobility, remarkably prevalent already, is soon expected to become a fact of life even in such traditional grow-your-own-talent industries as oil and steel. Says John F. Schlueter, executive director of the Association of Executive Recruiting Consultants: "Where executives have all been cut out of the same cloth, they are being criticized for it. My own feeling is that that will change. Cross-fertilization is going to become essential."

Beyond just hopping companies, hopping careers is also becoming acceptable. In this age of self-expression, it is now socially permissible

self-evaluation: your structural leadership profile*

The following twenty statements relate to your ideal image of leadership. We ask that as you respond to them, you imagine yourself to be a leader and then answer the questions in a way that would reflect your particular style of leadership. It makes no difference what kind of leadership experience, if any, you have had or are currently involved in. The purpose here is to establish your ideal preference for relating with subordinates.

The format includes a five-point scale ranging from "strongly agree" to "strongly disagree" for each statement. Please select one point on each scale and mark it as you read the twenty statements relating to leadership. You may omit answers to questions that are confusing or to questions that you feel you cannot answer.

	Strongly Agree	Agree	Mixed Feelings	Disagree	Strongly Disagree
1. When I tell a subordinate to do something I expect him to do it with no questions asked. After all, I am responsible for what he will do, not him.	(1)	(2)	(3)	(4)	(5)
2. Tight control by a leader usually does more harm than good. People will generally do the best job when they are allowed to exercise self-control.	(5)	(4)	(3)	(2)	(1)
3. Although discipline is important in an organization, the effective leader should mediate his use of disciplinary procedures with his knowledge of the people and the situation.	(1)	(2)	(3)	(4)	(5)
4. A leader must make every effort to subdivide the task of his people to the greatest possible extent.	(1)	(2)	(3)	(4)	(5)
5. Shared leadership or truly democratic process in a group can only work when there is a recognized leader who assists the process.	(1)	(2)	(3)	(4)	(5)

Continued on following page.

self-evaluation: your structural leadership profile (continued)

	Strongly Agree	Agree	Mixed Feelings	Disagree	Strongly Disagree
6. As a leader I am ultimately responsible for all of the actions of my group. If our activities result in benefits for the organization I should be rewarded accordingly	(1)	(2)	(3)	(4)	(5)
7 Most persons require only minimum direction on the part of their leader in order to do a good job.	(5)	(4)	(3)	(2)	(1)
8. One's subordinates usually require the control of a strict leader.	(1)	(2)	(3)	(4)	(5)
9 Leadership might be shared among participants of a group so that at any one time there could be two or more leaders.	(5)	(4)	(3)	(2)	(1)
10. Leadership should generally come from the top, but there are some logical exceptions to this rule.	(5)	(4)	(3)	(2)	(1)
11. The disciplinary function of the leader is simply to seek democratic opinions regarding problems as they arise.	(5)	(4)	(3)	(2)	(1)
12. The engineering problems, the management time, and the worker frustration caused by the division of labor are hardly ever worth the savings. In most cases, workers could do the best job of determining their own job content.	(5)	(4)	(3)	(2)	(1)

Continued on following page.

	Strongly Agree	Agree	Mixed Feelings	Disagree	Strongly Disagree
13. The leader ought to be the group member whom the other members elect to coordinate their activities and to represent the group to the rest of the organization.	(5)	(4)	(3)	(2)	(1)
14. A leader needs to exercise some control over his people.	(1)	(2)	(3)	(4)	(5)
15. There must be one and only one recognized leader in a group.	(1)	(2)	(3)	(4)	(5)
16. A good leader must establish and strictly enforce an impersonal system of discipline.	(1)	(2)	(3)	(4)	(5)
17. Discipline codes should be flexible and they should allow for individual decisions by the leader given each particular situation.	(5)	(4)	(3)	(2)	(1)
18. Basically, people are responsible for themselves and no one else. Thus a leader cannot be blamed for or take credit for the work of his subordinates.	(5)	(4)	(3)	(2)	(1)
19. The job of the leader is to relate to his subordinates the task to be done, to ask them for the ways in which it can best be accomplished, and then to help arrive at a consensus plan of attack.	(5)	(4)	(3)	(2)	(1)
20. A position of leadership implies the general superiority of its incumbent over his workers.	(1)	(2)	(3)	(4)	(5)

*This questionnaire is used with permission of the author, Dr. David R. Frew, associate professor of organizational behavior at Gannon College, Erie, Pennsylvania. The test appears in Dr. Frew's book, Management of Stress (Nelson-Hall, 1977).

structural followership profile

This section of the questionnaire includes statements about the type of boss you prefer. Imagine yourself to be in a subordinate position of some kind and use your responses to indicate your preference for the way in which a leader might relate with you. The format will be identical to that within the previous section.

	Strongly Agree	Agree	Mixed Feelings	Disagree	Strongly Disagree
1. I expect my job to be very explicitly outlined for me.	(1)	(2)	(3)	(4)	(5)
2. When the boss says to do something, I do it. After all, he is the boss.	(1)	(2)	(3)	(4)	(5)
3. Rigid rules and regulations usually cause me to become frustrated and inefficient.	(5)	(4)	(3)	(2)	(1)
4. I am ultimately responsible for and capable of self-discipline based upon my contacts with the people around me.	(5)	(4)	(3)	(2)	(1)
5. My jobs should be made as short in duration as possible, so that I can achieve efficiency through repetition.	(1)	(2)	(3)	(4)	(5)
6. Within reasonable limits I will try to accommodate requests from persons who are not my boss since these requests are typically in the best interest of the company anyhow.	(5)	(4)	(3)	(2)	(1)
7. When the boss tells me to do something that is the wrong thing to do, it is his fault, not mine, when I do it.	(1)	(2)	(3)	(4)	(5)

Continued on following page.

structural followership profile

	Strongly Agree	Agree	Mixed Feelings	Disagree	Strongly Disagree
8. It is up to my leader to provide a set of rules by which I can measure my performance.	(1)	(2)	(3)	(4)	(5)
9. The boss is the boss. And the fact that he has been promoted suggests that he has something on the ball.	(1)	(2)	(3)	(4)	(5)
10. I only accept orders from my boss.	(1)	(2)	(3)	(4)	(5)
11. I would prefer my boss to give me general objectives and guidelines and then allow me to do the job my way.	(5)	(4)	(3)	(2)	(1)
12. If I do something that is not right it is my own fault, even if my supervisor told me to do it.	(5)	(4)	(3)	(2)	(1)
13. I prefer jobs that are not repititious, the kind of task that is new and different each time.	(5)	(4)	(3)	(2)	(1)
14. My supervisor is in no way superior to me by virtue of his position. He simply does a different kind of job, one that includes a lot of managing and coordinating.	(5)	(4)	(3)	(2)	(1)
15. I expect my leader to give me disciplinary guidelines.	(1)	(2)	(3)	(4)	(5)
16. I prefer to tell my supervisor what I will or at least should be doing. It is I who is ultimately responsible for my own work.	(5)	(4)	(3)	(2)	(1)

scoring and interpretation

You may score your own leadership and followership styles by simply averaging the numbers included in parenthesis below your answers to the individual items. For example, if you scored item number one, "strongly agree," you will find the point value of "1" below that answer (Leadership Profile). To obtain your overall leadership style add all the numerical values associated with the twenty leadership items and divide by twenty. The resulting average is your leadership style. Followership is measured the same way, using the sixteen items contained within Part II of the instrument.*

		Interpretations	
Score	Description	Leadership Style	Followership Style
Less than 1.9	Very Autocratic	Boss decides and announces decisions, rules, orientation	Can't function well without programs and procedures. Needs feedback
2.0– 2.4	Moderately Autocratic	Announces decisions but asks for questions, makes exceptions to rules	Needs solid structure and feedback but can also carry on independently
2.5– 3.4	Mixed	Boss suggests ideas and consults group, many exceptions to regulations	Mixture of above and below
3.5– 4.0	Moderately Participative	Group decides on basis of boss's suggestions, rules are few, group proceeds as they see fit	Independent worker, doesn't need close supervision, just a bit of feedback
4.1– & up	Very Democratic	Group is in charge of decisions: boss is coordinator, group makes any rules	Self-starter, likes to challenge new things by himself

*It should be noted that scores on this instrument will vary depending upon mood and circumstances. Your leadership or followership style is best described by the range of scores from several different test times.

to pick up something new in mid-career. The rapid obsolescence of certain professions, the wholesale unemployment of highly skilled professionals, and the growing interest in generalists are all part of the phenomenon. So is our affluence. People can afford now to take a drop in salary for a while, or even forever, in order to work at a more satisfying career.

changing careers

Dr. Harry Levinson offers this advice to executives who want to take a different career direction:

Find a model. Look for someone you care to emulate, and find out how he got where he is, and what is involved in being there.

Supplement the consultation with vocational guidance if necessary. Your talents, skills, abilities, and preferences may be hidden to you. Check your local university's psychology department for reliable sources of counseling and testing.

Lay out a plan for self-development. Identify your goal and discover the steps that have to be taken to get there. Find out the formal and informal steps and list the alternatives. Include what you should read, what meetings you should attend, etc.

Persevere. The alternative, Dr. Levinson reminds us, is failure. Make the preparation stage enjoyable.

Watch Out for Promotions

Many executives, despite an outer image as a man of steel, cringe inwardly at the thought of assuming increased responsibility. Based on some deep fear of failure or inadequacy, such anxiety is a subtle killer because it is not one the executive is likely to admit to himself.

Further compounding the stress of promotions is the cultural problem known as status anxiety. Suddenly your old cohorts treat you differently. You are torn between the desire for power and the need for affection. The danger lies in trying to hold on to the old camaraderie and the new power at the same time. Bending over backward to be liked may undermine your position and make matters worse.

Each position of responsibility carries with it a certain image. As with any other change, this, too, can make the individual uncomfortable—beyond accommodating new ways of dressing and new places to eat. New techniques of organizing and communicating are called for, and these carry with them the anxiety of looking like an imbecile or failing utterly.

Perhaps the most frequent complaint associated with responsibility is the lack of concomitant authority. That is, people are often told to get a job done without being given the power to do it. This is especially lethal when one's performance is affected by the work of others over whom he has no authority. Dr. Levinson cites the case of a marketing coordinator who was expected to get six plant managers to use the same packaging for a particular product, but who had less authority in the company than any of the plant managers.

For these reasons many executives are shocked when their long-sought promotion turns out to be more anxiety producing than the pursuit of the position. Dr. Levinson's fundamental axiom is never to accept a promotion that requires you to behave differently from the way you like to act.

---

lessening the impact of relocation

Most companies dispense information, sympathy, and money to ease the pain of uprooted families. Take full advantage of these offerings.

Be alert to the needs of your children. Interestingly, younger children find moving easier than do teenagers, who tend to be more reliant on social ties.

Summer moves are harder on children, who have to find new friends without the structure of school. Investigate the schools in the new area. Here are some specific points to probe at a high school:

If the senior class has only 100–150 students, much valuable specialization will be missing. 300–500 is ideal at a three-year senior high school. Class size should not exceed 30.

A quality school will have one guidance counselor for every 250–300 students, and at least one career counselor.

A good school will have at least ten commendation winners under the National Merit Scholarship program, while an excellent school will have fifteen to twenty a year.

The list of courses should be extensive, with ample offerings in the sciences and languages, as well as advanced courses in the humanities.

In most upper-income suburbs, about 70 percent go on to college. But press for an answer to how many grads enter top schools.

Junior highs should have special provisions for slow learners and the very bright; elementary schools should have a classroom-size library with a full-time librarian, and a limit of 20 per class.

Allow three months or more for the implications of the move to be digested by the entire family.

Make sure you know what the company will pay for and what it won't. Larger companies, for example, will safeguard an executive by buying his house or by covering any loss on a sale. Compute your costs and make sure your allowance is realistic.

It is considered wiser to ask for a first-year bonus at the new location rather than a larger moving allowance.

Weigh the cost of moving in relation to any change in the cost of living your new location might demand.

Be sure to investigate the tax implications of your move.

Be careful of the hidden costs of moving—trips to house-hunt, closing costs on the sale of your house, redecorating, moving van, packing, etc.

> *Make at least two three-day visits in the new area. Start with an overview and narrow down to a specific town or neighborhood.*
> *Read the local papers. Check out the library, town hall, shops, food markets, and restaurants. Test the commutation time and comfort by yourself—don't take others' word for it.*
> *Ask yourself if you should relocate in the first place.*

women at work

It took a decade of federal legislation, relentless agitation from the women's movement, and drastic shifts in public opinion, but women are—at last—moving into the mainstream of corporate management. Women are making headway—slowly in the executive suite, faster at the lower rungs of middle management.

This remarkable social upheaval, like all changes, carries with it sources of destructive stress. Indeed, because it has occurred so suddenly and so massively, and because its implications resound throughout society, it could be the most significant challenge of all. Not just for the women, but for the men whose bastions are being penetrated. Both male and female executives should be aware of the unique set of psychological problems created by the new, rising managerial woman.

Sex consciousness and counterproductive attitudes are not likely to disappear overnight. If a male superior feels threatened by a competent woman's ability, he can create obstacles that neither government regulation nor common sense can overcome. Often such fear is unconscious, making it more insidious.

Getting in the door is easier than ever, but rising up the ladder is the real frontier. The middle-management level seems to be the most traumatic for both sexes. Women moving into middle management may meet resistance from male counterparts unenthusiastic about new and unusual competitors. Managers often will not dismiss an incompetent woman for fear of the Equal Employment Opportunities Commission, and there are some who are convinced that any woman who holds a managerial job owes it purely to the EEOC. However, a University of Southern California survey of companies that moved women into corporate positions formerly occupied by men reveals that almost all experienced fewer problems than either the men or the women had anticipated.

Discrimination is still rampant in many companies, especially above lower middle management. "I see ten- and fifteen-year women veterans in good staff line jobs still not being promoted," says management consultant Theodora Wells. "I see solid female professionals who should be prime candidates for upper middle management and would be if they were male. Companies feel free to play games with young

MBAs. But they won't spend the money to give their experienced women staffers what they need—accelerated growth in a controlled situation under the guidance of a male sponsor."

Sometimes recruitment is merely cosmetic, says Janet Jones, an executive director of Management Woman, Inc., a New York recruiter specializing in women. Companies may wish only to satisfy the government or the company president that they made the effort.

Behavior based on sex is a reality that government pressure and intellectual commitment can't easily erase. "I can remember, as a young product manager, going to the director of research and wanting to talk confidentially about a new product," recalls Diane Levine, staff vice-president at Continental Air Lines. "I went in, closed the door, and the guy couldn't even stay seated at his desk. He kept moving around the office until finally he went over and opened the door. Then he was able to sit down and talk. He was so concerned that someone might think something was going on behind closed doors!"

The Pressure to Excel

The pressure of being first adds an extra burden to newly arrived women. "If I were a male, I could probably make at least one small mistake without disrupting my career," says Jo Ann Fikes, one of the first female corporate lending officers at the United California Bank. "As a woman, I know there's no room for even one."

It is not paranoia that is giving women the attitude that they must perform at 300 percent efficiency at all times. A recent study found that top management generally accepted a certain male failure rate as a matter of course, but regarded female failure as an argument against further promotion. Says one female corporate president, "Really, what women are fighting for is the right to be just as mediocre as men have been."

Role Expectations

While many feel that women must resocialize themselves in order to succeed as executives, others point out that the extant male patterns may not be the healthiest—mentally or physically. No one knows which is more natural or which will produce the right combination of success and happiness.

Male social conditioning leads them unconsciously to expect something different from females. Yet they do demand businesslike behavior from anyone who seeks to achieve corporate goals. "In situations where men say, 'This is what I want and deserve' and get a yes or no, a woman's requests are treated as demands," says Sandra Kresch, vice-president at Booz, Allen & Hamilton, Inc., Chicago-based management consultants. "People are surprised and ask, 'Why is she such a hard-driving lady?'"

If a woman executive comes on strong, she risks alienating her male superiors. If she comes on soft, she convinces them that she lacks management qualities. This damned-if-you-do, damned-if-you-don't quandary can paralyze a woman and affect her health and career adversely.

Most experts believe that the woman executive's single greatest handicap is the lack of a role model. Dozens of little things that one must learn, men can find out by looking around them. Women have no one to copy.

Then there are other questions, such as, what to wear at each level? When does she start to call her boss by his first name? Who lights the cigarette? Who opens the door? Who enters the elevator first? With no one to emulate, many women run the risk of becoming imitation men.

Child care often determines the course of a woman's career, with many having to make key decisions around the availability of babysitters and qualified day-care centers. Even those, however, work well for 9-to-5ers, but not for an executive, who can't abruptly take off a few days when her child catches cold, or leave the office during a business emergency because she has to pick up her child. Certainly she can't do those things if she wants to advance.

Even the woman without children faces problems that men rarely faced: how to run both the household and the job, what to do about a promotion that would involve geographic separation, what happens emotionally when the wife's title or salary outranks the husband's?

Some companies have taken to hiring couples in order to avoid corporate rivalry and geographical problems. Many are even considering company-sponsored child-care centers.

Even when all the barriers to female advancement are down and the corporate world demands neither more nor less of women than it does of men, the woman who wants executive status will still pay a stiff price for it: the price men pay. Stress has no gender. The rate of stress disorders has already risen among corporate women, many of whom are developing heart trouble and ulcers, formerly the exclusive privileges of men.

Says Dr. Charles Winterhalter, medical director of Pitney-Bowes in Stamford, Conn.: "Women are getting coronaries as never before, but I can't say whether it's because they have been thrown into business situations with the same pressures as the men or whether some of it is due to the life-style that goes along with the situation, with smoking and drinking and other things. The alcohol problem is way up among women in the managerial levels, but I can't say whether that is due to stress or social environment."

Dr. Tobias W. Brocker, director of Menninger's Center for Applied Behavioral Science, feels that once women executives survive in the current, highly stressful period of being conspicuous exceptions in unfamiliar roles, they will probably stand the gaff better than men. "Women tend to have higher psychological and physical endurance for stress," he says. "They know more about their own feelings and it's easier for them to deal with emotions."

your best bet— live a balanced life

All work and no play not only makes Jack (or Jill) dull, it makes him (her) ill. Furthermore, it makes him (her) a lousy worker. The executive with an exaggerated sense of his own indispensability, or who harbors the erroneous notion that success requires 16-hour workdays, more often than not finds himself making mistakes, losing perspective, and otherwise defeating his own purpose—working effectively. The individual who paces himself, on the other hand, comes to work refreshed and alert, with new insights gained from having stepped back from the job. Like the well-paced distance runner, he will still be going at top efficiency when he reaches the wire.

"Some executives lack an internal governor for regulating the work-rest-recreation balance," states Dr. Benjamin Natovitz, director of medicine at Executive Health Examiners. "They deny fatigue and push themselves beyond reason. This is where stress sets in and the consequences of stress appear.... Unfortunately, I think that very few of us devote the insight and energy that we bring to furthering our business or professional careers to ourselves." A survey of 4000 executives found that less than 40 percent had a meaningful pastime.

There is sound physiological reasoning behind exhortations to lead a balanced life. "The body is not built to take too much stress always on the same part," writes Dr. Selye. "In stress research, we have found that, when completion of one particular task becomes impossible, diversion, a voluntary change of activity, is frequently as good as—if not better than—a rest. For example, when either fatigue or enforced interruption prevents us from finishing a mathematical problem, it is better to go for a swim than just to sit around."

Furthermore, it will help you work out the problem effectively. "A diversion into a substitute activity not only stimulates completion," writes Selye, "but it does so quite efficiently, and usually provides its own satisfaction."

———————————— **toward a healthier world** ————————————

In a very real sense, we have been a Type A society, aggressive, compet-itive, and oriented toward achievements that can be measured in num-bers like Gross National Product. In the sixties, the first generation to be endowed with a lifetime of material bounty said, in effect, thank you, but material affluence is not enough. On the heels of that impetu-ous protest came the reasoned voices of authorities—the physicians and researchers—who told us that our way of life was taking its toll on our minds and bodies. In this respect stress researchers like Hans Selye may ultimately be credited with opening the eyes of a nation and precipitat-ing a major historic transformation.

Perhaps the most encouraging development in the pursuit of a fuller life for everyone is that businessmen are now taking an active interest in the well-being of employees and themselves. American business has played a key role in making us the first nation to achieve virtually universal affluence. It might also help us become the first to achieve holistic health and a spiritual fullness.

———————————— **recommended reading: chapter 10** ————————————

Changing Organizations, Warren Bennis (New York: McGraw-Hill, 1966).

De-Managing America, Richard Cornuelle (New York: Random House, 1975).

Integrating the Individual and the Organization, Chris Argyris (New York: Wiley, 1964).

Management by Objectives, Stephen Carroll and Henry Tose (New York: Mac-millan, 1973).

Motivation and Personality, Abraham Maslow (New York: Harper Brothers, 1964).

Motivation to Work, Frederick Hertzberg (New York: Wiley, 1959).

New Patterns of Management, Rensis Likert (New York: McGraw-Hill, 1961).

Organization and Environment, Lawrence and Lorsch (New York: Irwin, 1965).

The Human Side of Enterprise, Douglas McGregor (New York: McGraw-Hill, 1960).

Toward a Psychology of Being, Abraham Maslow (New York: D. Van Nostrand, 1968).

index

263